Dedication

To all those who cope bravely with diabetes.
They teach me humility and understanding every day.

July 2013

To Yashoda with best wishes,

THE DIABETES ANSWER BOOK™

Practical Answers to More Than 300 Top Questions

David K. McCulloch

DAVID K. MCCULLOCH, MD

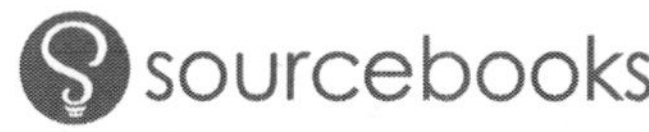

This book is not intended as a substitute for medical advice from a qualified physician. The intent of this book is to provide accurate general information in regard to the subject matter covered. If medical advice or other expert help is needed, the services of an appropriate medical professional should be sought.

Published by Sourcebooks, Inc.
P.O. Box 4410, Naperville, Illinois 60567–4410
(630) 961–3900
Fax: (630) 961–2168
www.sourcebooks.com

Library of Congress Cataloging-in-Publication Data

McCulloch, David K.
The diabetes answer book : practical answers to more than 300 top questions / David K. McCulloch.
p. cm.
Includes index.
1. Diabetes—Popular works. I. Title.
RC660.4.M375 2008
616.4'62—dc22

2008027159

Printed and bound in the United States of America.
POD 10 9 8 7

Contents

Acknowledgments

I am grateful to my agent, Jacky Sach, for giving me this opportunity.

As a medical student and young doctor in the 1970s, I was inspired and encouraged by two great mentors: Professor Ian W. Campbell in Edinburgh and Professor Robert B. Tattersall in Nottingham. They showed me how to make the complexity of diabetes accessible to people of all ages and in all walks of life. I have tried to follow their example of compassion and humanity in my clinical practice over the past thirty years.

In compiling this book, I am grateful to my colleagues and patients who supplied many of the questions and critiqued my answers to ensure that they were written in plain language: Dan and Rita Bockman, Lynn Briggs, Char Benedict, Mary Pat Bergin-Sperry, Meredith Cotton, Debbie Ciani, Monica Droker, Felipe Frocht, Annamarie Flott, Carol Freeman, Gage Foster, Kay Herndon, Patricia Heaven, Deborah Huang, Debra Hensler, Tenece Jones, Joan Kocher, Susan Kolberg, Dan Kent, Steve and Linda McDonald, Kelly McGraw, Janet Nolte, Mamatha Palanati, Vladimir Polyakov, Martha Price, Sue Ruedebusch, Sandy Randles, Nichole Richardson, Kathryn Ramos, Tim Scholes, Alan Searle, Rizwana Siddiqui, Lynda Sager, Betsy Schmidt, Wende Wood, Susan Weinstein, Lynn White, and Susan Whorton.

Finally to my editors at Sourcebooks, Sara Appino and Shana Drehs, for their careful attention to making this book as readable and useful as possible.

Introduction

To say that the management of diabetes has changed in the past thirty years is a major understatement. It has been transformed. When I became interested in diabetes as a medical student in Edinburgh in the 1970s, there were only two types of pill to help lower the blood glucose. The insulin we used contained impurities that could cause ugly scars where it was injected. Patients used large glass and metal syringes that had to be taken apart and boiled once a week to keep them clean. The needles were large and had to be sharpened on a Carborundum stone when they got blunt. The only way to have any idea what your blood glucose level was involved urinating into a test tube, adding a Clinitest tablet, and seeing what color it turned when it had finished boiling and frothing. While this exciting spectacle may have appealed to our inner alchemist, the information that it gave was about as useless as hanging seaweed out of the window and inspecting the color of that a few minutes later. People with diabetes lived in constant fear of passing out from low blood glucose levels (hypoglycemia) or of developing awful complications of their disease. The day-to-day burden on their lives was enormous.

The past three decades have seen many advances. There are now many different types of pill to help lower blood glucose and to protect the kidneys, heart, and blood vessels from the ravages of diabetes. We now use highly purified analogs of human insulin that can be delivered using disposable pens and tiny needles. You can carry little meters in your pocket that can give you an accurate blood glucose reading in a matter of seconds from just a drop of blood. Other tests allow us to know how well diabetes is being managed overall and how healthy the heart and kidneys are. Insulin pumps, inhaled insulin, continuous glucose monitors, pancreas and islet transplantation have all become realistic treatment options for some patients.

Yet people with diabetes still live in fear of passing out from hypoglycemia or of developing awful complications of their disease. The day-to-day burden on their lives is still enormous. The proliferation of new and alternative treatments and the blizzard of information and misinformation on the internet and other media make life more confusing than ever for people who have to live with diabetes.

In this book I will try to demystify diabetes and give you common sense answers to many of the questions that I get asked every day. I have divided the book into sections to make it easier for you to find answers on topics that you are interested in. If you don't find an answer to a question you have about diabetes, or if you want more detail about an answer that I have given, I invite you to write to me at the weblog that accompanies *The Diabetes Answer Book*, www.morediabetesanswers.com.

Some Questions Before We Start

- Am I a diabetic, or do I have diabetes?
- Should I say blood glucose or blood sugar?
- What is a hormone?
- What's the difference between a dietitian and a nutritionist?
- Can you make it understandable without dumbing it down?
- Why are drug names so confusing?
- Are the answers in this book only useful if you live in the United States?
- What if I still have diabetes questions after reading all these answers?

Am I a diabetic, or do I have diabetes?

I have many patients who say to me, "I have been a diabetic for fifteen years…" and then go on to ask their question. But when I speak to them or to any audience about diabetes, I never refer to them as being "a diabetic." I prefer to say "someone with diabetes." You may think this is a trivial distinction, but I don't. Many people, including me, are offended when they hear someone in crutches and leg braces being called "a spastic," and someone who has occasional brain seizures being called "an epileptic." As far as I am concerned, the diseases and problems that you have to deal with every day do not define who you are as a person. To me, the patients whom I try to help are all interesting and very different people with all sorts of jobs, families, hobbies, and stories to tell. They just happen to have diabetes as well. This is a significant burden to add to their lives, but it does not define who they are. Throughout this book I will try to give useful and practical answers to questions that you might have about having diabetes and living with diabetes, but I will not refer to you or anyone else as being a diabetic.

Should I say blood glucose or blood sugar?

This is a minor thing to make a fuss about. When patients say to me, "Why are my blood sugars so high in the morning, Dr. McCulloch?" they are being quite correct. But since I use the term so often throughout the book, I want to explain why I prefer to talk about blood glucose rather than blood sugar. Sugars are refined (or "simple") forms of carbohydrate. The basic building block of carbohydrates is a molecule with six carbon atoms joined together in a ring. Glucose is one example of a simple six-carbon sugar molecule. This is the form of sugar that floats around in your blood and gives energy to your muscles and brain and other parts of your body. There are other six-carbon sugar molecules, like fructose and galactose.

Table sugar is a larger molecule called sucrose, which is made up of joining a glucose and a fructose molecule together. Starches like bread, rice, potatoes, and pasta are more "complex" kinds of carbohydrate where hundreds of six-carbon sugar building blocks are joined together. Because I will be talking about different kinds of carbohydrates and sugars in answering questions about the food we eat, I am going to refer to the sugar that floats around in your blood (and causes so much frustration and stress to you!) by its proper name—blood glucose.

What is a hormone?

A hormone is a substance that is made in special cells in one part of your body and then gets pushed into the blood, where it travels to other parts of your body to have its effect. For example, special cells in the thyroid gland in your neck make thyroid hormones that get sent all over your body to help all your muscles and bones and nerves and other cells work properly. Groups of cells that make hormones are called endocrine glands, so your thyroid gland is an endocrine gland. Insulin is a hormone, so the pancreas is another endocrine gland. When your body does not make enough insulin or does not respond to it properly, it can lead to diabetes, so I will talk a lot about insulin in this book. I will also mention quite a few other hormones that affect your blood glucose.

What's the difference between a dietitian and a nutritionist?

Both of these terms are used for people who have special training to help you eat food that is healthy for you. Many people think that a "diet" always means you are being told to eat less so that you lose weight. Because of that, they imagine that a *dietitian* is someone who always wants you to lose weight. In recent years, people have started using the term *nutritionist* more often because it suggests, correctly, that these are people who think about how healthy the food is that you eat, not just how to help you eat less. Instead of being "put on a diet," you might be told that someone has been given a prescription for medical nutrition therapy. Whether I use the word *nutritionist* or *dietitian*, I am referring to people who can help you understand how to think about what you are eating and change it in ways that will keep you healthier and with blood glucose levels that are where you want them to be. When you are choosing a doctor, a nurse, or a nutritionist, there are two important things to look for. First, does this person really know a lot about diabetes? Second, is this person easy to get along with? Does he or she relate well to me and understand how to help me achieve my goals?

Can you make it understandable without dumbing it down?

That is definitely my plan in answering these questions. I have been talking to people with diabetes for over thirty years. Most of them are very smart and ask detailed and thoughtful questions. They deserve thoughtful answers that give as much detail as they need to understand it properly. Medical terminology can sound complicated and hard to understand. Lots of the words are really long and hard to pronounce. It is difficult to know what they mean unless you have a Latin dictionary! But it is usually easy to say the same thing in plain language. I have tried to do that as much as I can. Some people I work with are expert at talking in plain language and I have asked them to look over my answers and help me say it in a way that is easy to understand. That does not mean I will make an answer simpler than it really is. But I will try to use language that is easy to understand.

If you looked up what causes type 2 diabetes in a big medical textbook, you might get a sentence like this: *Type 2 diabetes occurs due to genetically determined amyloid deposition in the pancreatic islet cells, resulting in progressive deterioration in their capacity for insulin secretion.* You might read that and think, "Huh? I must be dumb, because I don't understand that." That is not true. "Medical speak" makes it sound really complicated, but it is possible to say all that stuff using words that most people can understand: *Insulin is a substance made in your pancreas in special cells called islet cells. When you inherit the genes for type 2 diabetes from your parents, these islet cells begin to fill up with strange stuff called amyloid. Over years, more and more amyloid clogs up the inside of your islet cells so that they make less and less insulin.* Putting it like that is not dumbing down the meaning, just making it easier to understand. I hope that this approach makes the answers more useful to you.

Why are drug names so confusing?

The chemical names for most drugs are really long, with lots of numbers and dashes that list every branch chain of the molecule. For example, there is a popular, long-acting kind of insulin. Its chemical name is 21A-Gly-30Ba-L-Arg-30Bb-L-Arg-human insulin, which is not very easy to remember! This usually gets shortened to another strange name called the generic name. The generic name for this insulin is glargine insulin. That is still not a very easy name to remember. Pharmaceutical companies use marketing companies and focus groups to find a catchy name that will appeal to the people they want to buy the drug. These are called trade names. The trade name of this popular insulin is Lantus, which is much easier to remember.

Here is another example. There is a class of drugs called phosphodiesterase inhibitors that can help men who have trouble getting an erection. This is a problem that worries a lot of men and may make them feel embarrassed or inadequate. The chemical name for one of those drugs is 1-[[3-(6,7-dihydro-1-methyl-7-oxo-3-propyl-1H-pyrazolo[4,3-d]pyrimidin-5-yl)-4-ethoxyphenyl]sulfonyl]-4-methylpiperazine citrate, but that isn't a very "sexy" name, if you'll pardon the pun! Even the generic name, sildenafil, doesn't sound very appealing. They wanted to come up with a name that would sound masculine, vigorous, healthy, confident, and powerful, and so they came up with Viagra. Now that sounds like a drug that will help erectile dysfunction!

It can get even more confusing once several different pharmaceutical companies all make the same drug. The actual drug name and generic names are the same, but they all have different trade names. A common drug to treat type 2 diabetes is metformin. It is sold under several different names (Fortamet, Glucophage, Glucophage XR, Glumetza, Riomet). In the answers in this book, I will give the generic name of a drug and then give one or two of the most common trade names, in brackets, afterward.

Are the answers in this book only useful if you live in the United States?

Not at all. I grew up in Scotland and worked as a doctor for many years in several cities in Scotland and England with people who had diabetes. Wherever you live around the world, you will have to deal with the same kinds of issues if you have diabetes. When I talk about blood glucose or cholesterol levels, I will give these in "American" units first and then give the "International" units in brackets afterward. I am sure that all of the books that I suggest are available outside the United States. The websites and other internet resources should also be available almost everywhere.

What if I still have diabetes questions after reading all these answers?

I hope that the answers in this book are detailed enough to help you. If you still find something confusing, or if you have follow-up questions, I invite you to send them to me on the weblog that I have set up to accompany this book. The address for that is www.morediabetesanswers.com. I will share my answers on the blog. I will also use the feedback you give me to improve the answers or add new answers to new questions if we do a second edition of *The Diabetes Answer Book.*

Part One:
The Big Picture

Chapter 1

Causes of Diabetes

- What is diabetes mellitus?
- What causes diabetes?
- What is insulin, and how does it work?
- What is insulin resistance?
- Is diabetes caused by having too little insulin or by being resistant to insulin?
- Can insulin resistance be treated?
- Is diabetes caused by eating too much sugar and junk food?
- Is diabetes caused by being overweight?
- Can stress cause diabetes?
- Why are so many people getting diabetes nowadays?
- Does diabetes ever go away on its own?
- Does diabetes "skip a generation"?
- How can I get diabetes if no one in my family has it?
- How does pregnancy cause diabetes that goes away after the baby is born?
- When is it helpful to measure the insulin level in a person's blood?
- What is C-peptide?
- When is it helpful to measure the C-peptide level in a person's blood?
- What is islet cell antibody (ICA)?
- What is glutamic acid decarboxylase antibody (GADA)?
- When is it helpful to measure ICA and GADA?
- When are genetic tests useful?

What is diabetes mellitus?

I hesitate to answer this question because you may find the answer so disgusting that you won't want to read the answers to any other questions! The history of diabetes is really fascinating. Back in ancient times, a few thousand years ago, doctors noticed that some people were struck down with a strange malady. In other words, they were sick for some unknown reason. They kept having to go to the bathroom to urinate, in other words "pee," all the time. It was as if their bodies had turned into water siphons or as if someone had left the faucet running. The Greek word for that was *diabetes.*

Now, these ancient doctors didn't have the fancy lab tests that we have today, but they did have smart brains and could use their own senses. They found that if they tasted the urine from these patients (that's the disgusting part), they could tell between two different kinds of diabetes. With some of these patients, the urine was insipid, meaning it didn't taste of anything much. They said that these people had *diabetes insipidus*. However the urine from some of their other patients tasted as sweet as honey. The Latin word for "honey sweet" is *mellitus,* so the doctors said that these people had *diabetes mellitus*. That term has "stuck" in the medical literature for a few thousand years and is still used today. For the rest of this book, I will simply use the term diabetes, but you'll know that I'm talking about the condition that causes "honey-tasting urine," or diabetes mellitus.

What causes diabetes?

If the blood glucose level in a person's body stays higher than normal, that person is said to have diabetes mellitus. Many things can cause this to happen. The main thing that keeps our blood glucose in the normal range is a hormone called insulin, which is made in the pancreas. The pancreas is a small organ in your abdomen, behind your stomach. The main job of the pancreas is to make chemicals (juices and enzymes) that help us digest the food we eat. The other job of the pancreas is to make hormones, including insulin. These hormones are made by little islands of cells in the pancreas known as islet cells.

When something happens that hurts either the pancreas or the islet cells inside it, then the body can't make enough insulin to keep blood glucose normal. And this causes diabetes. For example, if someone has pancreatic cancer and has surgery to take out the pancreas, that will cause diabetes. A condition called pancreatitis can also lead to diabetes. Pancreatitis is when a person's pancreas gets inflamed and swollen. Those are examples of something that hurts the pancreas itself. And if a person has inherited genes that cause the islet cells in the pancreas to stop working properly, that will also cause diabetes.

What is insulin, and how does it work?

Insulin is a hormone that's made in specialized cells in your pancreas. A hormone is a chemical substance that's made in one part of the body, gets released into the bloodstream, and is used by other organs in the body. The insulin hormone is needed so that the body's organs can use glucose for energy. Without insulin, or when insulin can't work well, glucose builds up in the blood and causes high blood glucose. The insulin hormone is a protein molecule. It has fifty-one smaller building blocks called amino acids. Insulin has two chains. The A-chain contains twenty-one amino acids, while the B-chain contains thirty amino acids. The two chains are linked together.

Although you don't need to know the chemical structure of insulin to be able to understand it and use it properly, you might be interested to see what it looks like. Later, I'll tell you how scientists have modified the chemical structure of the insulin molecule to

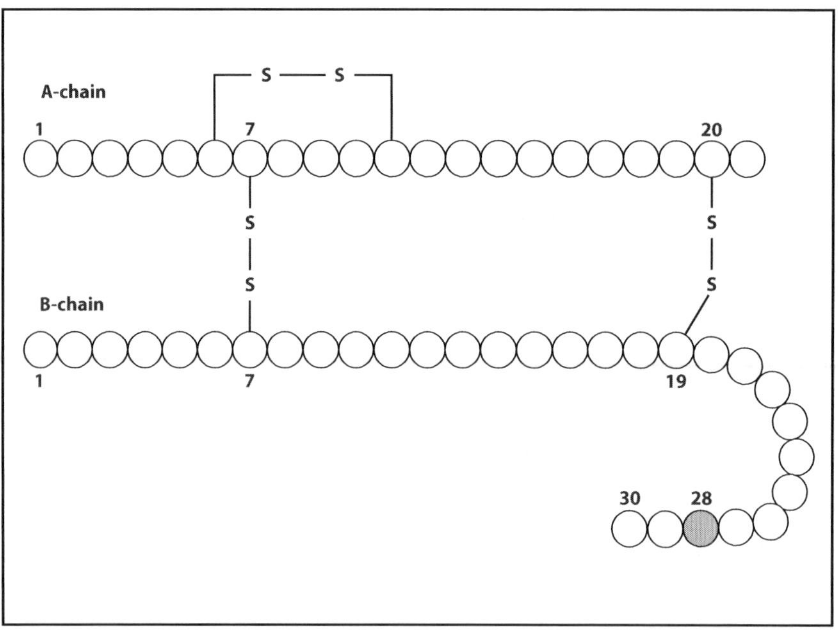

Figure 1: Chemical Structure of the Insulin Molecule

make newer kinds of insulin (called analogs) that work even better than the insulin made by the human body.

After the insulin molecule is made in the pancreas, it's released into the blood stream and travels to other organs in the body. When the insulin molecule arrives at an organ where it's needed, one end of the insulin molecule attaches itself to an insulin receptor (receiver) on the outside of the organ's cells. Think of it like this: insulin is like a key. The insulin receptor on the cell is like the lock. When the insulin key fits inside the receptor, it unlocks a door in the cell wall to let molecules of glucose enter that cell. This is what gives the cell energy. Our muscles are a good example of organs that need glucose for energy. Insulin allows glucose to enter the cells of our muscles to give us energy when we exercise. Other organs that need insulin in order to work are our fat cells and our liver cells.

Insulin does other useful things in our body. It helps us turn the food we eat into fat and protein. We can then store the fat to use for energy, and we use protein to build strong, healthy bodies. Insulin also helps us keep normal levels of fat in our blood stream.

What is insulin resistance?

Certain organs in our bodies need insulin to help them work. When the cells of those organs have trouble using insulin, we call it insulin resistance. Insulin receptors help our organs use insulin. Imagine a cell on an organ, such as a muscle. It normally has a thousand insulin receptors on its surface. These receptors are large chemical molecules formed inside the cells of our organs. They're designed to help our organs receive insulin molecules. Remember our lock and key analogy. The insulin is like the key, and the receptor is like the lock. The cells of our organs are constantly making new insulin receptors. The receptors are formed inside the cells, float up, and stick onto the outside of the cell surface. Then they come back inside the cell again.

When we exercise regularly, the cells in our bodies make more insulin receptors that float up and stick to the outside of the cells of our muscles and other organs. This makes our bodies better able to use insulin, and we become less insulin resistant. When we stop exercising regularly, the number of insulin receptors on the surface of our cells gets fewer and fewer over time. When the number of insulin receptors drops off, insulin can't unlock as many doors, and so less glucose can get into the cells. Sometimes when there are fewer insulin receptors around, our bodies respond by making more insulin.

Imagine we are in a group of one hundred people. The task of our group is to open a hundred doors of a house all at the same time. But there's a guard at each door that won't let us in. We probably won't be very successful. But if we are in a group of one thousand people, and we all rush those hundred doors at the same time, we have a better chance of getting in. That's what our bodies are trying to do when they make more insulin molecules. Our bodies hope that some of those insulin keys will open the locks to the cells of our organs.

There are other causes of insulin resistance. Sometimes insulin resistance is caused because the insulin receptor is the wrong shape or because the person has developed antibodies (chemical molecules that are made in the body) that sit on the receptor and block it so that insulin can't get in. Another cause of insulin resistance is high levels of other hormones in the blood that fight against the effects of insulin. For example, when a person is under a lot of stress, his or her body makes high levels of adrenaline, cortisol (a steroid hormone), glucagon, and growth hormone. These hormones do things that make it harder for insulin to work properly.

Is diabetes caused by having too little insulin or by being resistant to insulin?

People don't get diabetes unless their bodies make too little insulin. Even someone who is very resistant to insulin will have normal blood glucose levels if he or she can make enough insulin to overcome the resistance. Many people who are overweight have fewer insulin receptors on their cells than people who are thinner. But if the pancreas of an overweight person can keep making more and more insulin, he or she can overcome insulin resistance and keep the blood glucose normal. This is exactly what happens. When someone is very overweight and has normal blood glucose levels, then that person has much higher levels of insulin in his or her blood than a thinner person. Even while the insulin-making cells in the pancreas are slowly being destroyed, they might be able to make enough insulin to keep blood glucose levels normal. But only as long as the cells of the organs still have plenty of receptors on them. When the number of receptors on the cells drops off, the ailing insulin-making cells won't be able to make enough extra insulin to keep up. Finally, when the body stops being able to make enough insulin, it can't overcome insulin resistance any longer. That's when blood glucose levels will go up and lead to diabetes.

Can insulin resistance be treated?

Several things can improve insulin resistance. When you lose weight, your body will start to put more receptors on the surface of your cells, and you'll become less insulin resistant. As you start to exercise, your body will respond by putting more insulin receptors on the surface of your cells, and you'll become less resistant to insulin. If insulin resistance is caused by stress, then it will improve when you find ways to lower your stress. If you have to take high doses of corticosteroid drugs (to treat asthma or arthritis, for example) it can cause tremendous insulin resistance. If another way can be found to treat your asthma or arthritis (or another condition), and you can lower the dose or stop taking the steroid drug, then the insulin resistance will improve. There are also some drugs you can take to improve insulin resistance. These include metformin and a group of drugs called thiazolidinediones (or glitazones). I'll talk about these drugs in more detail in response to other questions in the book.

Is diabetes caused by eating too much sugar and junk food?

No. This is what we call an "old wives' tale": a story that mothers and grandmothers used for many years to scare children into eating a healthier diet. Don't get me wrong; I don't think that eating a lot of junk food is good for you. There are all sorts of reasons why it's healthier to eat food with more fiber and vitamins and less sugar, sodium, caffeine, and fat than what you get in most "junk food." But no food by itself will ever cause diabetes. Many teenage athletes can eat lots of candy, pizza, and potato chips, and yet they stay lean, muscular, fit, and glowing with health. Part of the reason is that they're young and their bodies are growing. They also burn up all those extra calories when they exercise.

Most of us find, as we get older, that if we keep eating the same kind of food and in the same amount that we ate as teenagers, we quickly feel dreadful. We gain weight, and we get stiff and sluggish. The key thing is to balance how much we eat and how much we exercise. If we take in more calories than we can burn up, day after day, then we'll gain weight. The body can't tell where calories come from. Whether we eat "healthy" calories or "junk" calories, we'll gain weight if we take in more of them than we can burn up through exercise and other activities.

If your body is unable to make lots and lots of insulin, and you eat lots of refined carbs, like candy and regular pop, you'll certainly have a higher blood glucose for the next few hours than someone who can crank out enough insulin to handle the "junk food" load. But eventually, your blood glucose will return to normal. While it's certainly easier for the body to deal with food that has more fiber and less sugar than most junk food, eating junk food does not directly cause diabetes. Diabetes happens when a person isn't able to make enough insulin to keep their blood glucose normal.

Is diabetes caused by being overweight?

Being overweight doesn't directly cause diabetes. However, it does cause you to become more and more resistant to the effects of insulin. No matter how overweight you are, you won't develop diabetes if your body can keep making enough insulin to overcome that resistance. The problem is that all of us, as we get older, start to make less and less insulin. But this process starts earlier in life and progresses faster if someone has the genes for type 2 diabetes. That's why some people who are overweight in their twenties or thirties still have normal blood glucose levels. But as they get older, their blood glucose levels will start to go up. Unless they do something to lower their insulin resistance (for example, eat less, exercise more, and lose weight), they'll develop impaired glucose tolerance and then diabetes.

Can stress cause diabetes?

When I tell you that the answer to this is "no," many of you may disagree vigorously! Many people are convinced that some form of stress caused their diabetes. In fact, they're sure of it. Their diabetes came on immediately after a car accident or a divorce or after being laid off from a job. There are several reasons why these kinds of traumatic and stressful events can cause diabetes to "appear."

Imagine that you have inherited the genes for type 2 diabetes. Remember that in type 2 diabetes, the cells that make insulin are programmed to stop working properly. A substance called amyloid becomes deposited inside those cells and over time, they make less and less insulin. You feel fine and your blood glucose levels are normal because, even though you're making less insulin than you used to, you still make enough to keep glucose going from your blood into your cells. Now, if you get really stressed, your body will respond by pushing out high levels of adrenaline, cortisol (a steroid hormone), glucagon, and growth hormone. These hormones do things that make it harder for insulin to work properly. So at this point, the amount of insulin that your body makes is not enough. Your blood glucose levels rise. You feel tired, thirsty, and sick. You go in to see your doctor, who tells you that you have diabetes.

The close association between the stressful event and the onset of diabetes makes it seem like a clear cause-and-effect. In truth, the stressful event simply exposes the fact that your body can't make as much insulin as it needs. The same thing happens with people who are diagnosed with type 1 diabetes. It often seems that their diabetes came on when they were stressed out. Maybe they were studying for school exams and then got a sore throat and chest infection. It seems like those things "caused" their diabetes. But in fact, the immune system in those people had been quietly destroying their insulin-producing cells for several months or years before they got stressed with exams and then an infection. Again, stress can expose or "unmask" diabetes by increasing the amount of insulin the body needs. If your body cannot respond to this demand, then diabetes develops.

Why are so many people getting diabetes nowadays?

You often hear in the media that there is an epidemic of obesity and diabetes, especially in the United States. There are several reasons for this. Lifestyles have changed dramatically in the past few decades. Most people used to have jobs that required physical labor (like farming). They cooked most of their own meals. They had far fewer "labor-saving" electronic devices, and didn't have the hassles of dealing with those devices, like having to remember PIN numbers and passwords.

Nowadays, many of us have desk jobs, so we aren't as physically active. Many of us don't have time to cook, so we eat out more often. And we're more stressed then ever, dealing with all the usual concerns about work, family, and friends. Not only that, we have to deal with an ever-growing number of gadgets. So we get less exercise, eat out more, and are more stressed. The food industry has responded to our need for quick, tasty food by making high fat, high calorie, sugary, salty food that's more delicious, easier to get, and more affordable than ever. And it comes in bigger and bigger sizes.

Of course, we should all take personal responsibility for what we eat and how we spend our time, but it can be really hard. Plate sizes and portion sizes are much bigger nowadays. Not many of us are able to only eat part of what's on our plate and throw the rest away or save it for another meal. We have less time to plan ahead to make sure we have healthy food at home. And we have less time to make sure we get exercise every day. A combination of all these things is making more and more of us overweight or obese. That extra weight causes insulin resistance. If your body isn't able to make enough extra insulin to overcome that resistance, then you'll get diabetes.

Does diabetes ever go away on its own?

It is incredibly rare for diabetes to ever go away on its own, although there are certain situations when it seems like it has gone away for good. Imagine that your body makes less insulin than it should. It can make just enough to keep your blood glucose normal, if it isn't asked to work too hard. If you eat a healthy diet, keep your weight down, exercise regularly, and stay happy and stress-free, then your blood glucose levels will stay normal. But imagine that something changes in your life to make you need much more insulin. You get sick and need to be put on high doses of corticosteroid drugs (like Prednisone). Suddenly you develop diabetes. If you can come off of the steroids, your diabetes might go away completely. Or imagine that you've gained a hundred pounds over many years and now have diabetes. If you could dramatically and permanently lose all of that weight (as a result of gastric bypass surgery, for example), then your diabetes might seem to go away completely.

Pregnancy is another example of something that can lead to diabetes. When a woman gets pregnant, she needs to make more insulin to meet the extra demands of her growing body and growing baby. If she isn't able to increase the amount of insulin her body makes, she'll get diabetes during her pregnancy. This is called gestational diabetes. Once the baby is born and her body returns to normal, her diabetes might go away completely.

In all of the situations described above there's a chance that diabetes will come back. As we get older, we gradually make less insulin, and many of us also become more resistant to insulin, especially if we gain weight or have more aches and pains and stresses in our life. So people who had diabetes when they were on steroids when they were younger and women who had diabetes while they were pregnant have a higher chance that the diabetes will come back later in their lives.

Does diabetes "skip a generation"?

This is another "old wives' tale" that many people believe. While it's true that diabetes may skip a generation now and then, it doesn't happen often enough to be predictable.

Imagine that a man comes from a family where several people, including him, have diabetes. If that man marries a woman who has no diabetes in her family and they have children, it's possible that none of their children will have diabetes. Some of their children might inherit a susceptible gene from their father, but a more powerful protective gene from their mother. In this case, these children won't get diabetes any time during their lives. However, if one of these non-diabetic children grows up and has children of their own, they might pass on the susceptible gene that they got from their father. If their partner doesn't pass on a protective gene, then their children may get diabetes. In that situation, there was diabetes in both the grandparents and the grandchildren but not the generation in the middle. So you can truly say that diabetes "skipped" a generation. Although it happens like this from time to time, it isn't something that you can rely on when making decisions about having children and their likelihood of getting diabetes.

How can I get diabetes if no one in my family has it?

It's perfectly possible to have no diabetes in your family and still get diabetes or have children that do. We all carry thousands of different genes, some of which protect us against diabetes while others put us at some risk. In a family where no one has had diabetes for as long as anyone can remember, you can assume that there are many more protective genes being passed on than susceptible ones. It's possible that two parents with no family history of diabetes could each pass on a susceptible gene instead of a protective gene to their child. In that case the child could get diabetes even though there was "no diabetes in the family."

Another factor to remember is lifestyle. Some families may carry genes that put them at risk for developing type 2 diabetes. But if the members of those families have very active and healthy lifestyles (working at a job involving physical labor, eating healthy food, exercising a lot, and not getting overweight, for example), then they will never get diabetes. If they have children who move to the city, have stressful desk jobs, eat too much, don't exercise, and gain weight, then those children may get diabetes even though there was "no diabetes in their family."

How does pregnancy cause diabetes that goes away after the baby is born?

When a woman is pregnant, her body needs to make enough insulin to support her extra weight and her growing baby. By the time a woman is in her last three months of pregnancy, her body will need to make between three and four times as much insulin as it did before she became pregnant. If her body isn't able to increase the amount of insulin to meet the demand, then her blood glucose will rise, and she'll develop diabetes. This is known as gestational diabetes.

Most pregnant women can't tell if they've developed diabetes. After all, feeling tired, thirsty, and going to the bathroom more often are all part of being pregnant, even for women with normal blood glucose levels. That's why we've started to test women for gestational diabetes during the first half of their pregnancy. If a woman is diagnosed with gestational diabetes, her health-care team will help her learn to keep her blood glucose levels as close to normal as possible. She'll learn to make different food choices, and she might take pills or insulin.

If blood glucose levels are too high during pregnancy, the baby might be born too early. The baby's lungs might not be fully developed. Or the baby might be born with a blood glucose level that's too low. There's also a chance that the baby could be born with birth defects. After the baby is born and the woman's body returns to its normal size and weight, her diabetes will usually go away. However, women who had gestational diabetes are much more likely to develop type 2 diabetes later in life. About half of all women who had gestational diabetes develop type 2 diabetes within ten years after their babies are born. This time, though, the diabetes doesn't go away. Usually women who develop gestational diabetes have the genes for type 2 diabetes in their family. Even before they got pregnant, their body wasn't able to make as much insulin as it should. The extra demand for insulin that the pregnancy caused "unmasked" their insulin deficiency.

When is it helpful to measure the insulin level in a person's blood?

It's rarely helpful to measure the amount of insulin in a person's blood. Suppose there are two people with the same normal fasting blood glucose (less than 100 mg/dL.) But if we measure the amount of insulin in their blood, we find that one of them has a much higher insulin level than the other. What does that tell us? It tells us that the person with the higher insulin level is more resistant to insulin than the other person. The person who's resistant to insulin needs to put out more insulin in order to keep blood glucose levels normal. Maybe the person with the higher insulin level is overweight or more stressed, or maybe there's another reason for the insulin resistance. Measuring the insulin level in a person's blood does not help us to decide what to do for him or her.

One of the problems with measuring insulin in the blood is that it can change so quickly from minute to minute throughout the day. Insulin levels change depending on when you last ate, what you ate, when you last exercised, and how stressed you are. Although some doctors like to measure insulin levels and make decisions based on the results, it rarely gives us useful information that we can't get in other ways.

What is C-peptide?

There are a couple of steps to making insulin inside your pancreas. The first step is that your pancreas makes a big molecule called proinsulin. Then, when your pancreas is ready to release insulin into your bloodstream, it splits proinsulin into two new molecules. One of them is insulin. The other molecule is called the connecting peptide, or C-peptide for short. C-peptide is released into your bloodstream every time you secrete insulin. In fact, the pancreas releases an equal amount of C-peptide molecules as it does insulin.

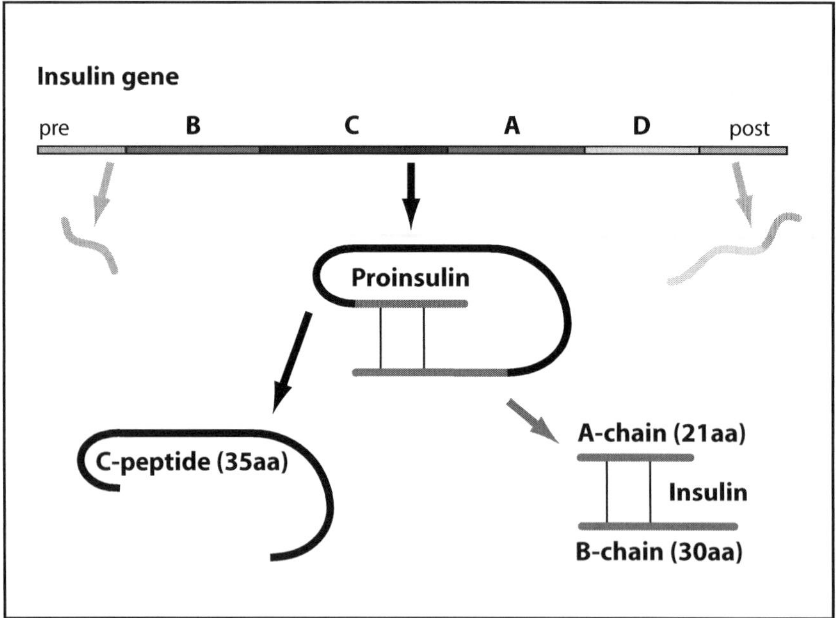

Figure 2: Relationship between Proinsulin, C-peptide, and Insulin

When is it helpful to measure the C-peptide level in a person's blood?

When people with diabetes take insulin shots, they only take insulin, not C-peptide. If we measure the insulin level in the blood of people who take insulin, we can't tell how much of that insulin they made in their own bodies and how much came from their insulin shots. But if we measure how much C-peptide is in the blood of someone with diabetes, we know it only came from the person's own pancreas. Because the body always releases the same amount of insulin as C-peptide, we can also tell how much insulin in the blood came from the person's own pancreas.

There are a few situations when it's helpful to know whether someone with diabetes is able to make any insulin from his or her own pancreas. In order to find out, we can stimulate the pancreas to push out as much C-peptide as it can by giving the person a shot of a hormone called glucagon. Or we can measure the C-peptide when the person's blood glucose level is above 200 mg/dL (or 11.1 mmol/L). If someone with diabetes can't make any C-peptide under those circumstances, it tells us that that person can't make any insulin either. It tells us that that person has complete insulin deficiency. People who have complete insulin deficiency are at a higher risk of making ketones if they don't get enough insulin. Ketones happen when the body can't turn glucose into energy and starts burning fat stores instead. This can lead to a life-threatening condition called diabetic ketoacidosis. Some insurance companies will only cover the cost of an insulin pump for people who are "C-peptide negative." In other words, for people who are completely unable to make any insulin in their own bodies and are at a higher risk of getting ketoacidosis.

What is islet cell antibody (ICA)?

Islet cell antibody (ICA) is an antibody aimed at the cells in the pancreas that make insulin. These insulin-making cells are called islet cells. If we find ICA in someone's blood, it tells us that the person's own immune system is making antibodies that are acting as if some part of the islet cell was a "foreign invader." It's too complicated to simply say that the antibodies are "attacking" the pancreas. The parts of the immune system that do most of the attacking are other cells (like lymphocytes) that release chemicals that can kill the islet cells. ICA is an autoantibody, meaning that it's aimed at part of our own body.

There are many different kinds of islet cell antibodies and different lab tests that can find them. About 70 percent or more of people with type 1 diabetes will have ICA that can be found in their bloodstreams at the time they are first diagnosed with type 1 diabetes. However, months and years later, the ICA may disappear from their bloodstreams. Why? Because after all of the insulin-making islet cells have been destroyed, there isn't anything left for the immune system to attack. It stops making antibodies to fight against it. The same thing happens when you get a virus, such as a head cold or the flu. While you're sick, your body makes lots of antibodies to fight that particular virus. But once it's been destroyed and you're feeling well again, the amount of antibodies your body made to fight against that virus falls to very low levels.

What is glutamic acid decarboxylase antibody (GADA)?

Glutamic acid decarboxylase antibody (GADA) is an antibody that the body makes to target a particular enzyme inside the insulin-making islet cells of the pancreas. It's an even more sensitive autoantibody than ICA. Over 80 percent of patients with type 1 diabetes will have GADA in their bloodstream when they are first diagnosed.

When is it helpful to measure ICA and GADA?

There are several times when measuring ICA and GADA can be helpful. If I see a child or a teenager who is overweight and has diabetes that can be controlled by a better diet, more exercise, and by taking pills to treat type 2 diabetes, I'll often check for ICA and GADA to make sure he or she doesn't have type 1 diabetes. If tests show that there's ICA or GADA the blood, it means the person does, in fact, have type 1 diabetes. In this case, I advise the patient to start taking insulin right away, even though the person could "get away with" using pills for several weeks or months. The reason for this is that, by using insulin in the early stages of type 1 diabetes, we can slow down how fast the rest of the person's insulin-producing cells are destroyed. This makes diabetes easier to control for the first several years. If someone with type 1 diabetes is treated with pills, it will speed up the rate at which the rest of the insulin-producing cells are destroyed.

If I see an older patient who has type 2 diabetes that doesn't seem quite typical, I'll also check for these antibodies. For example, maybe the person wasn't overweight when diagnosed. Or maybe the person had been losing weight even after starting pills that usually work well for type 2 diabetes. If the test finds either ICA or GADA, or both, in that person's blood, then I know that he or she has type 1 diabetes, and I advise the person to start on insulin right away.

It's also possible to check for ICA and or GADA in the non-diabetic children or siblings of someone with type 1 diabetes. The presence of these antibodies makes it more likely that those non-diabetic relatives have an autoimmune destructive process going on in their own bodies and may develop type 1 diabetes in the future. At the present time, there are no effective treatments to prevent such a person from getting diabetes. But this is a very active area of research that may help us to prevent type 1 diabetes in the future.

When are genetic tests useful?

At the present time, genetic testing is only used for research. Human Leukocyte Antigen genes that can make the immune system "misfire" (discussed in the next chapter) might tell us if someone is at risk of developing type 1 diabetes. But these genes are actually quite common. Millions of people carry at least one gene that makes them susceptible for diabetes, and yet they will never get diabetes. Sometimes, when two parents both have type 1 diabetes, they ask to have genetic tests done to see how big the risk is for their children developing diabetes. Genetic testing can give some idea of the future risk but can't say for sure. Even among genetically identical twins, if one of the twins develops type 1 diabetes, the chance that the other twin will develop type 1 also is less than half. But if the twin has type 2 diabetes, the chance that the other twin will get it too is higher, but it's still not 100 percent. In the future it may be possible to make more accurate predictions about lifetime risk of diabetes through genetic testing, but we're not at that point yet.

Chapter 2

Types of Diabetes

- How many types of diabetes are there?
- My doctor says I have "secondary" diabetes. What does that mean?
- What is impaired glucose tolerance?
- Does starting insulin make me a type 1 diabetic? Can you change from one type to another?
- What genes cause type 1 diabetes?
- What genes cause type 2 diabetes?
- What is type one-and-a-half diabetes?
- Can sixty-year-olds get "juvenile" diabetes?
- Can ten-year-olds get type 2 diabetes?
- Does it matter what type of diabetes you have?
- What is polycystic ovarian syndrome (PCOS)?
- What is the connection between PCOS and diabetes?
- Can a person carry the genes for both type 1 and type 2 diabetes?
- If I have type 1 diabetes, how likely is it that my children will get it?
- If I have type 2 diabetes, how likely is it that my children will get it?

How many types of diabetes are there?

The two most common types of diabetes happen when the insulin-making cells inside the pancreas are either destroyed or stop working properly. The rest of the pancreas still works normally, making other hormones and chemicals to help with digestion. But it can't make any, or enough, insulin to keep blood glucose normal. These types of diabetes are called type 1 and type 2.

Type 1 diabetes is a genetic disorder. It is also known as an autoimmune disease. This is because in type 1 diabetes the person's own immune system slowly destroys all the islet cells in the pancreas that make insulin. This can take many months or years to happen. During this time, the person feels fine. But when enough insulin-producing islet cells have been destroyed, the person will suddenly develop severe signs of diabetes. Type 1 diabetes is not common. Only 5 percent of all people with diabetes have type 1. But it's a serious condition. People with type 1 diabetes need to take insulin shots and closely monitor blood glucose levels in order to stay alive and healthy.

Type 2 diabetes is also a genetic disorder. In type 2 diabetes, the cells in the pancreas that make insulin are genetically programmed to stop working properly. A substance called amyloid gets deposited inside those cells and, over time, they make less and less insulin. In type 2 diabetes, the insulin cells are destroyed more slowly than they are in type 1 diabetes. Usually the pancreas of a person with type 2 diabetes is still able to make some insulin, even years after he or she was diagnosed with diabetes. It's just that the pancreas can't make enough insulin to keep blood glucose normal.

Although we still put people into one category or the other as either type 1 or type 2, we're still learning about diabetes and what causes it. In the future, as we learn more about the specific genes involved, it's likely that we may find there are many more types of diabetes.

My doctor says I have "secondary" diabetes. What does that mean?

When a person gets diabetes because of another illness, we call it secondary diabetes. The diabetes only happens because of the other condition. For example, if a person has surgery to remove the pancreas, then it will cause secondary diabetes. Conditions that destroy the pancreas, such as pancreatitis or cystic fibrosis, can cause secondary diabetes. Too much iron in the body, a condition called hemochromatosis, can also damage the pancreas and cause secondary diabetes. Certain kinds of tumors, like those in the adrenal gland or the pituitary, can cause the body to make too much corticosteroid hormone or too much growth hormone. These hormones prevent insulin from working properly and that can cause secondary diabetes.

What is impaired glucose tolerance?

Normal glucose tolerance is when a person's blood glucose stays in the normal range all the time. The fasting blood glucose (the blood test done first thing in the morning before a person eats anything) is always less than 100 mg/dL (or 5.6 mmol/L) in someone with normal glucose tolerance. If someone's fasting blood glucose stays between 100 and 125 mg/dL (5.6–6.9 mmol/L), then he or she is said to have impaired fasting glucose or impaired glucose tolerance. But if a person's fasting blood glucose is always over 125 mg/dL (or 6.9 mmol/L), then that person has diabetes. If the cells in the pancreas that make insulin are slowly destroyed by either a condition such as pancreatitis or by deposits of amyloid building up inside of the cells, then the person will begin to develop impaired glucose tolerance. If the destruction of the insulin cells goes on long enough, the person will move from impaired glucose tolerance to diabetes.

Does starting insulin make me a type 1 diabetic? Can you change from one type to another?

No. Even though everyone with type 1 diabetes needs to take insulin, a lot of people with type 2 diabetes eventually need to take insulin, too. With type 1 diabetes, the cells that make insulin usually get destroyed quite quickly. It takes much longer in type 2 diabetes for the cells that make insulin to stop working properly. Almost everyone with type 2 diabetes can make some insulin, even after having diabetes for thirty years or more. Some people with type 2 diabetes never need insulin. But about a third of people with type 2 diabetes eventually reach the point where the amount of insulin their bodies make isn't enough to overcome insulin resistance. So taking insulin shots is a good option for them. This doesn't mean that they've become type 1.

What genes cause type 1 diabetes?

Human beings have twenty-three pairs of chromosomes inside the nucleus of all of our cells. Each chromosome contains hundreds or thousands of different genes. We each inherit one set of chromosomes from our mother and another set from our father. There are a number of genes clustered together on chromosome number 6 that affect how the cells in our immune system work. Those cells include white blood cells and cells in our lymph nodes. These cells roam around the body looking for "foreign invaders" (like viruses and bacteria) and then work together to destroy them.

Some people inherit genes in the HLA (Human Leukocyte Antigen) region of chromosome 6 that make their immune system "misfire" sometimes. When those people encounter a "foreign invader" in their bodies (and again, it might be a bacterium or a virus or possibly even an unusual type of food), the cells in their immune systems begin attacking the insulin-producing cells of the pancreas as if they were foreign. When our immune system starts attacking part of our own body, we call it an autoimmune attack. If the autoimmune attack keeps going and growing in force, then it can end up destroying the insulin-producing cells completely, and that causes type 1 diabetes.

Interestingly, the genes that cause type 1 diabetes are quite common. Even though fewer than one out of a hundred people will get type 1 diabetes during their lifetime, more than ten times that number carry at least one of the genes that make them susceptible to the autoimmune attack that causes type 1 diabetes. When someone has a gene that makes him or her susceptible, it means it puts that person at risk for getting the disease. But most of us also have genes that protect us from getting type 1 diabetes. People have a mixture of susceptible genes that put them at risk and other genes that protect them. Whether you develop type 1 diabetes during your lifetime or not depends on a couple of things. It depends on whether you have more susceptible genes than protective ones. And it depends on whether or not you get a certain virus, bacterium, or other "foreign invader" that causes your immune system to misfire.

What genes cause type 2 diabetes?

We know less about the specific genes that cause type 2 diabetes than we do for type 1 diabetes. There are probably dozens of different genes that can work together in combination to affect your chances of getting type 2 diabetes. Some families have an unusual kind of type 2 diabetes that starts in childhood. This used to be called Maturity Onset Diabetes of the Young (MODY). In the past twenty years or so, scientists have found that these families have a single type of genetic defect that causes some of the family members to get type 2 diabetes early in life. While this teaches us a lot, it's clear that the more common forms of type 2 diabetes have lots of genes involved, many of which have not yet been identified. Those genes might affect how well the insulin-producing cells in your pancreas work and whether or not they will start failing at an early age. Other genes might affect how many insulin receptors you can produce on the surface of your muscle cells and fat cells or how well those receptors work.

What is type one-and-a-half diabetes?

This is an odd term that you may hear from time to time. When someone gets diabetes later in life, people might assume that person has type 2 diabetes. But maybe that person isn't overweight. And maybe that person is eating healthy foods, getting exercise, and taking all of his or her pills properly. But that person still ends up needing to take insulin. Some people say that this kind of person doesn't fit the picture for typical type 1 diabetes. But that person doesn't fit the picture for typical type 2 diabetes either. So often you'll hear people say the person has "type one-and-a-half" diabetes. I think that this kind of term simply shows that we still don't know enough about the genes that lead to diabetes to be able to classify it properly.

Can sixty-year-olds get "juvenile" diabetes?

Yes, they can. That's why we've stopped using the terms "juvenile-onset" and "maturity-onset" to describe types of diabetes. As a doctor, I've seen many examples of people in their sixties, seventies, and even eighties coming down with signs typical of type 1 diabetes. These patients were a normal weight and then suddenly started losing weight. They also started getting thirsty, tired, and urinating a lot. By the time they were diagnosed, they had to go into the hospital with a life-threatening condition called diabetic ketoacidosis. All of these signs combined suggest that these people had severe (almost total) insulin deficiency, meaning their bodies were making little or no insulin. Those patients of mine needed to treat their diabetes with insulin from the very start and were never able to come off it again. These older patients all had the same signs and symptoms that are typically seen in children with type 1 diabetes.

What's the explanation? It's likely that, although they had gone through their lives carrying at least one gene that put them at risk for developing type 1 diabetes, that gene never got "triggered." Maybe they never got exposed to a particular "foreign invader," such as a virus, bacterium, strange food, or whatever. Or maybe they'd been exposed to a few things during their life that caused their immune system to "misfire" slightly, but never enough to drive their immune system into a continuous attack. Whether someone develops type 1 diabetes at all, and when in his or her life that happens, clearly depends on how many of his or her genes are protective and how many are susceptible. But it also depends on how many "triggering" events he or she was exposed to over a lifetime.

Can ten-year-olds get type 2 diabetes?

Yes, they can. This is something I'm seeing more and more often nowadays, because so many more young people are overweight and don't exercise. If someone has inherited the genes for type 2 diabetes, that means that his or her body will gradually make less insulin as he or she grows older. Exactly how soon this person's ability to make insulin starts to get weaker depends on the genes that the person inherited and the kind of lifestyle he or she leads. People who stay active and keep their weight down can keep making enough insulin to keep their blood glucose normal well into adulthood. However, children who don't get regular exercise and gain weight can start to show signs of insulin resistance at an early age. If a child's body can't make enough insulin to overcome that resistance, then that child will develop type 2 diabetes.

Does it matter what type of diabetes you have?

Sometimes it isn't possible to be absolutely sure if someone has type 1 or type 2 diabetes. How healthy you stay during a lifetime with diabetes doesn't depend on whether you have type 1 or type 2 diabetes. What matters more are the choices you make and the way your diabetes fits into the rest of your life. I'll go into this in more detail as I answer questions later in this book. However, there are some situations where it really does help to know if someone has type 1 or type 2 diabetes. An example that I see quite often is a teenager who is a bit overweight and has just been diagnosed with diabetes. When he or she stops eating so much candy and regular pop and starts exercising more regularly, his or her diabetes becomes quite well controlled. Sometimes the teenager will have been started on a pill like metformin or a sulfonylurea, drugs that we use to treat type 2 diabetes. The teen may even be doing fine on it. So it's as though the teen has type 2 diabetes.

However, I still worry about whether the teen might have type 1 diabetes instead of type 2, and here's why. In type 2 diabetes, the insulin-producing cells are slowly being destroyed by getting amyloid deposited in them. But in type 1 diabetes, the destruction is usually faster and is caused by the person's own immune system attacking his or her pancreas. If I can be sure the teen has type 1 diabetes (and the antibody tests that I described in the last chapter can prove someone has type 1 diabetes), I would advise this teenager to start taking insulin right away, even though he or she could "get away with" using pills for several weeks or months. The reason for this is that, by using insulin in the early stages of type 1 diabetes, we can slow down how fast the rest of the insulin-producing cells are destroyed. This makes diabetes easier to control for the first several years. If someone with type 1 diabetes is treated with pills, it speeds up how fast the rest of his or her insulin-producing cells are destroyed.

What is polycystic ovarian syndrome (PCOS)?

PCOS is a condition that's quite common in women: they have irregular menstrual periods; their ovaries might stop making eggs; they become infertile, gain weight, and can develop lots of hair in places where women usually don't (such as on the face, chin and upper lip). The ovaries of these women can get very large and develop cysts (pockets of fluid) in them. Many women with PCOS also have trouble with greasy skin and acne. The skin around their arm pits and groins can become thickened, darker, and velvety to the touch (a condition called acanthosis nigricans).

What is the connection between PCOS and diabetes?

The specific genes that cause PCOS haven't been found yet, but there's probably an overlap between those genes and the genes that cause insulin resistance and type 2 diabetes. PCOS often happens in women who come from families that have type 2 diabetes. The key feature that PCOS and type 2 diabetes have in common is insulin resistance. Treating the insulin resistance in women with PCOS can help improve fertility and decrease the amount of hair and acne on their skin.

Can a person carry the genes for both type 1 and type 2 diabetes?

Yes. Although we haven't been able to identify all the genes involved, we know that the genes that cause both type 1 and type 2 diabetes are common in the general population. Most of the time, people will get the same kind of diabetes as their parents or other members of their families. But it's also quite possible for someone to come from a family that has a history of type 2 diabetes and still get type 1.

If I have type 1 diabetes, how likely is it that my children will get it?

The risk of developing type 1 diabetes depends on several factors, including your ethnicity, family history, and what particular genes you inherit. Let's say that you're of European ancestry (an ethnicity with a fairly high risk for developing type 1 diabetes). There are two main genes that increase your risk (DQB*0201 and DQB*0302), and one gene that protects against type 1 diabetes (DQB*0602). Imagine that neither of your parents and none of your siblings have diabetes. If you inherited two DQB*0201 genes, one from your mother and the other from your father, your risk of getting diabetes in the future would be about 1 in 350. If you inherited two DQB*0302 genes, then your risk would be higher (about 1 in 60), and if you inherited one of each (let's say a DQB*0201 from your mother and a DQB*0302 from your father), your risk would be higher still (about 1 in 25).

If you were lucky enough to inherit a DQB*0602 from either parent, then your risk falls to about 1 in 1,500. But if either of your parents or any of your siblings already have type 1 diabetes, the chance that you'll develop it too goes up a lot. For example, if you have inherited two of the DQB*0201 gene and either of your parents or any of your siblings have type 1 diabetes, your chances of getting it too go from 1 in 350 to 1 in 20. With two of the DQB*0302 gene, your chances go from about 1 in 60 to 1 in 10. And if you inherit one of each (DQB*0201/DQB*0302), your chances go from 1 in 25 to 1 in 4. What this tells us is that people who have type 1 diabetes in their immediate families must carry additional genes that we have not yet identified. These genes, along with DQB*0201 and DQB*0302, put people at an even greater risk for type 1 diabetes.

If I have type 2 diabetes, how likely is it that my children will get it?

If you or your partner has type 2 diabetes, then the chance that any of your children will develop diabetes in the future is quite high (at least 1 in 4 in some families). The chances for getting type 2 diabetes are higher in families from certain ethnic backgrounds, including Native Americans, Pacific Islanders, Hispanics, and African Americans. But the chances that someone in a family will get type 2 diabetes are harder to figure out than for type 1. Although we have found some specific genetic mutations that we can link to rare forms of type 2 diabetes, we know much less about the genes that increase a person's chances of getting the more common forms of type 2 diabetes.

Chapter 3

DIAGNOSIS

- My doctor says I have diabetes, so why don't I have any symptoms?
- What are the symptoms of diabetes?
- If I think I might have diabetes, what are the best screening tests to get?
- Who should be screened for diabetes?
- What is prediabetes ?
- What is the metabolic syndrome?
- What is the body mass index (BMI)?
- How do you know if you are normal weight, overweight, or obese?
- How can I tell if I have type 1 or type 2 diabetes?
- What is a normal blood glucose level?

My doctor says I have diabetes, so why don't I have any symptoms?

None of the symptoms of diabetes is specific for diabetes. In other words, there are other things that can cause those symptoms. If diabetes comes on slowly and your blood glucose gradually gets higher and higher over many years, you may not notice that you are feeling more tired than you used to. Maybe you assume it is just "old age" or that you are working too hard. You start having to go to the bathroom more often but assume it must be your prostate (if you are a man) or just a "weak bladder." You notice that you are drinking more cups of coffee or tea or water than you used to, but you shrug it off. You are just thirsty. It feels good to gulp down liquid when you are really thirsty. It is no big deal. In fact, you may think that it is no wonder that you are going to the bathroom so often to urinate since you are drinking so much liquid. Maybe you noticed that you were losing some weight but were quite pleased about that. Perhaps you assumed that it was because you were eating less due to stress from overwork. It is estimated that between four and eight million people in the United States may have diabetes right now but don't know it. This is one of the reasons why it is a good idea to screen people for diabetes.

What are the symptoms of diabetes?

When the blood glucose level gets too high, it can cause many symptoms. However, if the rise in blood glucose came on very slowly, you may not even have noticed the symptoms, or you may have thought they were due to something else. All of the symptoms can be caused by other things, but when several of these symptoms occur together, you should certainly think that you might have diabetes and should get yourself tested. When your blood glucose level gets high, your kidneys try to get rid of the glucose, and so going to the bathroom for excessive amounts of urination is the commonest symptom of diabetes. Since this gets rid of lots of extra water out of your body, you end up getting dehydrated and feeling very thirsty as a result. Funnily enough, many people are not surprised that they are going to the bathroom a lot. They assume that it is because they are drinking so much extra fluid that they need to go to the bathroom so much (rather than the other way around).

Diabetes can also affect your vision. Even though you will not notice any change in the size of your eyes, the inside of your eyeball swells with extra fluid. The hard lens inside the eyeball also begins to swell with extra fluid, but it takes much longer for the lens to swell or to shrink when the glucose levels change; and so sometimes the lens is too big, and sometimes it is too small for the size of your eyeball. This causes blurred vision. Sometimes people are so troubled by this that they go to their eye doctor and end up getting new prescriptions for glasses or contact lenses to compensate. If you do this before you realize you have diabetes and then get treatment to bring your blood glucose levels back to normal, then you will be annoyed that you spent all that money on new eyewear. Your new glasses or contact lenses will no longer work for you once your blood glucose levels are back close to normal and your eyeballs and lenses have returned to their normal size.

Some people also feel incredibly tired when they are developing diabetes. They may feel very hungry and may be losing weight no matter how much they eat. This is especially likely with type 1 diabetes, where your body makes so little insulin that you can't prevent fat and protein being broken down in your body. If the diabetes goes undiagnosed for even longer, you may feel drowsy and nauseated. Some people end up being taken to the hospital because they are so weak, or may even have passed out into a coma. When diabetes comes on more slowly, you may not notice any symptoms at all. Sometimes it is diagnosed when you go to see your doctor for another problem, such as erectile dysfunction or numbness in the feet. The high blood glucose can also make you at higher risk for getting certain types of infection such as yeast infections in your groin, penis, or vagina.

If I think I might have diabetes, what are the best screening tests to get?

To diagnose diabetes officially, you need to have your blood tested two separate times. If your blood glucose is taken after a ten-hour overnight fast and is higher than 125 mg/dL (6.9 mmol/L) on two occasions, then you have diabetes. If your blood is drawn at another random time (such as after a meal or in the middle of the afternoon) and is higher than 200 mg/dL (11.1 mmol/L) on two occasions, then you have diabetes. Also, one fasting value of over 125 mg/dL and one random value of over 200 mg/dL mean that you have diabetes. It used to be common for people to be given an oral glucose tolerance test (OGTT) to diagnose diabetes. To do this, you have to fast overnight, get your fasting blood glucose taken, and then drink 50–100 grams of glucose drink all at once (or within a minute or two). The blood glucose is then measured every half hour for the next two or three hours. If the fasting value is above 125 mg/dL, the peak is over 200 mg/dL, and the value at two hours is over 140 mg/dL (8.9 mmol/L), then you have diabetes.

Oral glucose tolerance tests are mostly only used to diagnose gestational diabetes nowadays or for research purposes. Some people use glycosylated hemoglobin (or hemoglobin A1c or HbA1c) to help screen for diabetes. I will say more about this important blood test in answer to other questions. HbA1c measures the average of the blood glucose levels in your blood over the past eight to twelve weeks. The higher your blood glucose gets, the more of your hemoglobin gets converted to HbA1c. For people who do not have diabetes, only 4 to 6 percent of hemoglobin is HbA1c. While it is not used as part of an official way to diagnose diabetes, if you have a HbA1c of 7.0 percent or higher, it is very likely that you will be found to have diabetes when you get your fasting or random blood glucose levels measured.

Who should be screened for diabetes?

The American Diabetes Association recommends that all adults over the age of forty-five should get a fasting blood glucose measured. A normal result is under 100 mg/dL (5.9 mmol/L). If this is the result you get, then you will be advised to get it repeated in three to five years. If your result is above 125 mg/dL (6.9 mmol/L), then you should have the test repeated within a week or two. If it is above 125 mg/dL on a second test, then you have diabetes. If your fasting blood glucose is between 100 and 125 mg/dL (or if the first test was over 125 mg/dL but the second one was below 125 mg/dL), then you have impaired glucose tolerance and are at risk of getting diabetes in the future. You will be advised to change some things in your lifestyle (by modifying what you eat and how much you exercise, for example) and will be asked to get your fasting blood glucose repeated every year.

Certain groups of people are at higher risk of getting type 2 diabetes, and they are often screened at earlier ages and more often. Certain ethnic groups (Native Americans, Pacific Islanders, Hispanics, and African Americans), people who have a family history of type 2 diabetes, and women who have had gestational diabetes are all at higher risk of getting diabetes.

What is prediabetes?

This term is used a lot these days, but I am not sure how useful it is. It can easily be misused. The term has become popular in the media and with drug companies who make drugs that might delay the onset of diabetes. Labeling people as having prediabetes certainly gets their attention! It suggests that we have a perfect crystal ball and can know ahead of time that someone is going to get diabetes. Once you know that someone has diabetes, you can certainly look back and say that, during the time before he or she got diabetes, he or she had "prediabetes." I suppose you could also say that while we are alive, we are all in a state of "predeath." The term prediabetes implies that we can identify people and know for sure that they are going to develop diabetes in the future. If people have a strong family history of diabetes and have been tested and were found to have impaired glucose tolerance, then they are certainly at much higher risk of getting diabetes in the future unless they can change something. But it is presumptuous to say that they have "prediabetes."

What is the metabolic syndrome?

People with certain physical characteristics and laboratory abnormalities are at higher risk of developing heart disease and diabetes. These abnormalities often cluster together. They include obesity (especially carrying too much weigh around your middle, called central obesity), hypertension (high blood pressure), high cholesterol and triglyceride levels in the blood, high uric acid levels in the blood, and insulin resistance. If you have one or more of those things, it is a good idea to get your fasting blood glucose checked every year, since you are at a higher risk of developing diabetes.

Some doctors think we should be taking waist measurements in our patients to make a more formal diagnosis of the metabolic syndrome, but they don't agree about which combinations of things you need to have in order to give someone that label. I must say that I do not routinely do waist measurements on my patients. It is incredibly difficult to do it accurately. The measurement varies depending on where around the body you wrap the tape measure and how relaxed they are, how big a breath they take, and whether or not they suck in their stomach. So if you do it several times on the same person, you can get very different results, and if two different people measure it on the same person, they may not agree either. I do not find that it is helpful to me or to my patients to label them as having the metabolic syndrome, but if I see someone who is overweight and has one or more of the other things mentioned above, then I test his or her blood glucose.

What is the body mass index (BMI)?

The body mass index has become the international standard way to describe how appropriate someone's weight is. It takes into account your height as well as your weight. This makes good sense. The ideal weight for someone who is four feet eleven inches tall is obviously less than the ideal weight for someone who is six feet ten inches tall. The formula is a little difficult for most of us to grasp (especially Americans who are used to thinking in terms of pounds rather than kilograms and feet and inches rather than meters). Your BMI is your weight (in kilograms) divided by your height (in meters) that is then squared. I am six feet tall and weigh 180 pounds. So my weight in kilograms is 180 divided by 2.2 (there are 2.2 pounds in a kilogram) or 81.8 kg. Six feet tall is 72 inches tall. There are 2.54 centimeters to an inch, so six feet works out to 1.83 meters. If I multiply that number by itself (or "square" it), I get 3.35. So 81.8 divided by 3.35 gives me a BMI of 24.4. If that is too complicated to do, there are many tables and calculators that do the calculation for you.

How do you know if you are normal weight, overweight, or obese?

If your BMI is under 18.5, you are underweight. If your BMI is between 18.5 and 24.9, this is considered to be an ideal normal weight range for your height. If your BMI is between 25 and 29.9, you are overweight. Anyone with a BMI over 30 is considered to be obese. Doctors used to use the term "morbid obesity" to describe people with a BMI over 40, but since some people find this term to be offensive and unhelpful, we now define three levels of obesity. Class I is 30–34.9; Class II is 35–39.9; and Class III is 40 or above. The risks to your future health go up as your BMI goes up, so this is a good thing to know about yourself.

How can I tell if I have type 1 or type 2 diabetes?

I mentioned in response to other questions that there are two antibodies that can be measured in your blood that tell if you have an autoimmune process destroying the insulin-producing cells in your pancreas. Those are islet cell antibody (ICA) and glutamic acid decarboxylase antibody (GADA). If you have high levels of one or both of those antibodies in your blood, then you have type 1 diabetes. About 90 percent of people with type 1 diabetes will have one or both of these antibodies present in their blood when they are first diagnosed, but over time, the level of these antibodies goes down until they can't be detected at all. And at least 10 percent of people with type 1 diabetes do not have ICA or GADA in their blood.

So the presence of ICA and GADA means you do have type 1 diabetes, but the absence of them does not necessarily mean that you don't. There is no test that says, "You definitely have type 2 diabetes." Some doctors measure insulin levels or C-peptide levels, but these do not tell if you have type 1 or type 2 diabetes. They simply tell that your body is still able to produce some insulin of its own at this time. That can be true if you have type 2 diabetes but can also be true in the first few months or years of having type 1 diabetes.

What is a normal blood glucose level?

The glucose level in your blood goes up and down all day long, whether you have diabetes or not. It is usually at its most stable and lowest level when you wake up in the morning and before you have eaten anything. The normal range for this fasting blood glucose is between 70 and 100 mg/dL (3.9–5.9 mmol/L).

Your blood glucose goes up after you eat food. How high it goes up and how fast it goes up depends on how much you eat and what type of food you eat. Carbohydrate (especially "simple" or refined carbohydrate like sugar, candy, and regular pop) can be absorbed very quickly and will push your blood glucose up quickly and to high levels for a few minutes at least.

For someone without diabetes, it is unlikely to ever get above 160 mg/dL (8.9 mmol/L). If it ever gets above 200 mg/dL (11.1 mmol/L), then you should have it checked a second time because you may have diabetes. Your blood glucose goes up with food, goes down when you exercise, usually goes up when you are stressed, and goes down when you relax. So even if you do not have diabetes, your blood glucose may go up and down between 70 and 160 mg/dL (3.9–8.9 mmol/L) throughout the day.

Chapter 4

PREVENTION

- What can I do to prevent myself from getting diabetes?
- What can I do to prevent my kids from getting diabetes if I have type 2 diabetes?
- Can improving your diet and doing more exercise really prevent type 2 diabetes?
- Are there drugs that can prevent type 2 diabetes?
- What can I do to prevent my kids from getting diabetes if I have type 1 diabetes?
- If I have type 1 diabetes, should my kids get tested for ICA and GADA?
- If I am pregnant and have diabetes, what can I do to make sure my baby stays healthy?

What can I do to prevent myself from getting diabetes?

It is a tired old joke to answer this question by saying, "Choose your parents wisely!" Obviously you are stuck with who you have as parents, and so your genetic risk is already set for you. As I will discuss in answer to another question, there are no effective ways to prevent someone from getting type 1 diabetes at the present time. But if you are at risk for getting type 2 diabetes (and really all of us are at some risk of getting type 2 diabetes when we get older), the best way to prevent it is to live a healthy life. Eat a healthy balance of types of food. Keep your weight close to ideal. Get regular exercise. Find time to do things that are relaxing and fun. Don't smoke. Don't drink alcohol to excess.

What can I do to prevent my kids from getting diabetes if I have type 2 diabetes?

The main thing you can do is to advise your kids to live a healthy lifestyle. If they are at higher risk of getting type 2 diabetes because it runs in your family, then you should suggest that they get screened for diabetes at an earlier age than is usually recommended (so even earlier than starting at age forty-five).

Can improving your diet and doing more exercise really prevent type 2 diabetes?

It really can. There was a landmark study published a few years ago called the Diabetes Prevention Program (DPP) that looked into this. In this study, researchers followed over 3,200 people with an average age of fifty-one. They were all obese (the average BMI was 34.1 kg/m2), and all of them had impaired glucose tolerance. Many of them came from high-risk ethnic groups, so they were at really high risk of developing type 2 diabetes in the following five years.

They were randomly placed into one of three groups. The first group was given general advice about healthy diet and exercise but got no extra help or support. They were what is called the "control group." Another group got the same advice but was also started on a pill called metformin, which can make your body respond better to insulin (so it reduces insulin resistance). The third group was given much more support and encouragement to eat healthier types and amounts of food and to exercise more. The goal for this group was to reduce their weight by 7 percent and to do at least thirty minutes of moderate exercise (like brisk walking) at least five days out of every seven (so a total of at least 150 minutes of exercise per week).

When they were evaluated three years later, 29 percent of those in the control group had already developed type 2 diabetes. Only 22 percent of those taking metformin had developed diabetes, but the most impressive result of all was that only 14 percent of those who improved their diet and did more exercise had developed diabetes. I find these results very encouraging. Let's talk about the weight loss first. If you are already overweight or obese, you may feel discouraged and think that you will have to lose a hundred pounds or more in order to reduce your chances of getting diabetes. But the DPP showed that if you can just change your eating habits enough to decrease your weight by 7 percent, you will dramatically reduce your risk of getting diabetes. That means if you weigh two hundred pounds, you need to lose fourteen pounds and keep it off. If you weigh three hundred pounds, you need to lose at least twenty-one pounds and keep it off. I am not suggesting that this is easy, but it is a much more reachable goal than most people think.

With exercise, some people who are overweight or obese get discouraged, because they think they will need to wear ugly spandex outfits and be embarrassed at the gym for hours on end in order to get the benefits of exercise. But the DPP showed that if you can just make sure you get at least thirty minutes of moderate exercise five days out of seven and keep this up for at least three years, then you will reduce your risk of getting diabetes by a lot. Regular exercise like this will also reduce your risk of heart disease, high blood pressure, and depression, so there are lots of benefits.

Are there drugs that can prevent type 2 diabetes?

As I mentioned in answer to the last question, taking metformin also reduced the risk of getting diabetes in the DPP. Several other drugs have also been shown to reduce the risk of diabetes. Acarbose, orlistat, and a class of drugs called thiazolidinediones (sometimes called TZDs or glitazones) have all been shown to reduce the future risk of getting type 2 diabetes. These drugs can all be used to treat people who already have type 2 diabetes.

There are a couple of important points to remember when thinking about using a drug to prevent diabetes. First, it is unclear whether these drugs prevent diabetes or simply delay it by a few years. That might still be worth while, but then again, it might not. If you take a drug that is expensive and may have unpleasant or dangerous side effects and it only delays the onset of your diabetes by two or three years, I am not sure that is a wise choice for you.

The other thing to remember is that all of these drugs are much more effective if you are also improving your eating and doing more exercise. I wish the DPP had included a fourth group that was supported to eat less and exercise more but also took metformin. I think the results would have been even more impressive, with less than 10 percent developing diabetes in the next three years and beyond. But that is just my guess. In order to know for sure, you really have to design a well-controlled, randomized trial.

What can I do to prevent my kids from getting diabetes if I have type 1 diabetes?

There is no safe and approved treatment to prevent type 1 diabetes. Some studies have shown that babies who are breast-fed are slightly less likely to get type 1 diabetes than babies who receive formula based on cow's milk. There has also been a lot of research trying to identify which non-diabetic relatives of people with type 1 diabetes are at the greatest risk of getting diabetes by doing genetic tests and also by measuring the level of islet cell antibody (ICA) and/or glutamic acid decarboxylase antibody (GADA).

We know that type 1 diabetes is usually caused when your own immune cells attack the insulin-producing cells in your pancreas. We also know that we can detect those antibodies months or even years before diabetes will develop. We can even measure how much insulin someone is able to make, and we can follow this over time to see if they make less and less insulin. The problem is that there are no effective ways to stop the autoimmune destruction that is going on. At least none of the treatments are considered safe to use in the long term.

There was a hope a few years ago that treating these ICA-positive, non-diabetic relatives with high doses of the vitamin nicotinamide might delay or prevent diabetes from developing, but that was proved to be wrong when it was tested in a properly designed, randomized trial. Researchers have also tried giving those relatives insulin (either by injection or by mouth) in the hope of stopping or slowing down the autoimmune process.

Again, the results from these trials have not been encouraging so far. It probably would be possible to stop the autoimmune process if we used high enough doses of powerful immunosuppressive drugs (the kind of drugs that are used to prevent the rejection of organ transplants), but these drugs have so many side effects when they are used for years on end that I fear the side effects of the treatment would be worse than getting diabetes and dealing with that. This is a very active area of research, however. I am optimistic that some safe and effective treatment will be found in the future to slow down or stop the autoimmune process that causes type 1 diabetes.

If I have type 1 diabetes, should my kids get tested for ICA and GADA?

Several major universities around the world are conducting research to identify children at risk for developing type 1 diabetes in the future. Some of them are also testing drugs to try to slow down or stop the process that will cause diabetes to develop. As I said in answering the last question, the results from these trials have been disappointing so far, but other studies are underway. If you wish to participate or to find out more, you can get information from the Juvenile Diabetes Research Foundation (www.jdrf.org) or from the American Diabetes Association (www.diabetes.org).

If I am pregnant and have diabetes, what can I do to make sure my baby stays healthy?

Most women with diabetes who get pregnant have perfectly healthy babies. Obviously if you are pregnant, then there are a number of things to do whether you have diabetes or not. You should get a check up with your health care team as early in your pregnancy as possible to check on your blood pressure and other signs of general health. You need to eat a healthy diet and take vitamins. The biggest worries related to diabetes are that if your blood glucose levels are too high during the pregnancy, then both you and your baby can have problems.

Ideally, if you have diabetes and are planning to get pregnant, you should try to get your blood glucose as well controlled as possible before you even get pregnant. A high blood glucose during pregnancy can cause the baby to put on a lot of extra weight. A bigger baby is harder to deliver. Also, if a baby is large, it may cause you to go into labor early, and so the risk of a premature baby is higher. Premature babies have a harder time breathing. Also, there is a risk that your baby can develop significant low blood glucose levels (hypoglycemia) in the first twenty-four hours or so after delivery.

Since your baby does not have diabetes and has a pancreas that is developing inside you while you are pregnant, high blood glucose levels can cause the baby's pancreas to put out high levels of insulin. Once the baby is delivered, those high insulin levels can push the baby's blood glucose down below normal, and that can cause problems including epileptic seizures.

For all of these reasons, you should see your health care team as early in your pregnancy as possible and stay in close contact with them during pregnancy, delivery, and afterward. There is a very slightly increased risk that your baby will have congenital malformations (birth defects) because you have diabetes, but this risk is much lower if you keep your blood glucose levels near normal and get regular checkups during your pregnancy.

Chapter 5

CURE

- How close are we to curing diabetes?
- What is a pancreas transplant?
- Who should get a pancreas transplant?
- What is the difference between a pancreas transplant and an islet cell transplant?
- Who should get an islet cell transplant?
- What are stem cells?
- Will stem cells cure diabetes?
- What is an artificial pancreas?
- Would an artificial pancreas cure diabetes?
- Does gastric bypass surgery cure type 2 diabetes?

How close are we to curing diabetes?

Let's make sure we have the same definition of "cure." For me, people with diabetes will consider themselves cured of diabetes if their blood glucose stays in the normal range no matter what they eat and without them having to think about it. That is the lucky position that people are in if they don't have diabetes. They don't need to remember to eat at particular times. They don't need to worry that their blood glucose will go too low if they sleep in, exercise too much, or forget to eat. Everything takes care of itself. By contrast, people who have diabetes have to pay attention to a whole lot of things all day, every day, in order to keep their blood glucose close to normal.

There are two main approaches to go about trying to cure diabetes. The first approach is to develop cells that will replace the insulin-producing cells that have been destroyed or that are functioning poorly. The options are pancreas transplants, islet cell transplants, or stem cell transplants. The second approach is to develop an artificial pancreas. This would involve a continuous blood glucose monitor that was connected to an insulin pump, so that whenever your blood glucose went up, the glucose monitor would detect this and tell the insulin pump how much insulin to give you to bring your blood glucose back down. Tremendous progress has been made in many areas of research in the past decade that is putting us much closer to a cure for diabetes than ever before.

What is a pancreas transplant?

When you think about someone getting an organ transplant, you usually think that your old and defective organ will be removed and that a new one will be put into your body in the same place as the old one was. After all, that is what we do if the battery in our car dies. We take out the old one and put a new one back in the same place. But there are several reasons why that is not what is done if you get a pancreas transplant.

First of all, you should remember that for most people who have diabetes, their own pancreas is still functioning almost perfectly. Over 99 percent of the pancreas is still working just fine. Your pancreas is lying up in your abdomen behind your stomach and attached to part of your intestines called the duodenum. The pancreas is a soft, squishy organ that weighs about 100–200 grams. It makes several pints of digestive juices and enzymes every day that it squirts into your guts to help you digest your food. You would not want a surgeon to remove that if it is working just fine. The only part that is not working is the little islands of cells scattered throughout your pancreas. You have between one and two million of these islets (named after the doctor who discovered them as the Islets of Langerhans). If you removed them all and piled them up, that pile would weigh only 1–2 grams. You could fit it on your thumbnail. So if you get a pancreas transplant, the surgeon will leave your own pancreas where it is.

Your new pancreas will come from an organ donor who has died. This pancreas has to be kept cold and treated with nutrients and brought to where it is going to be transplanted as quickly as possible. The new pancreas is removed from the donor along with a "collar" of the duodenum where it was attached to the donor's gut. The surgeon will place the new pancreas in your pelvis and attach it to your bladder by stitching the collar of the duodenum to the wall of the bladder. The surgeon connects blood vessels to the new pancreas so that it gets a supply of nutrients to keep it healthy.

Although this may seem an odd place to put the new pancreas, it makes a lot of sense when you think about it. Remember, the new pancreas is also spending 99 percent of its time and effort making digestive juices and enzymes. If those enzymes leaked into your

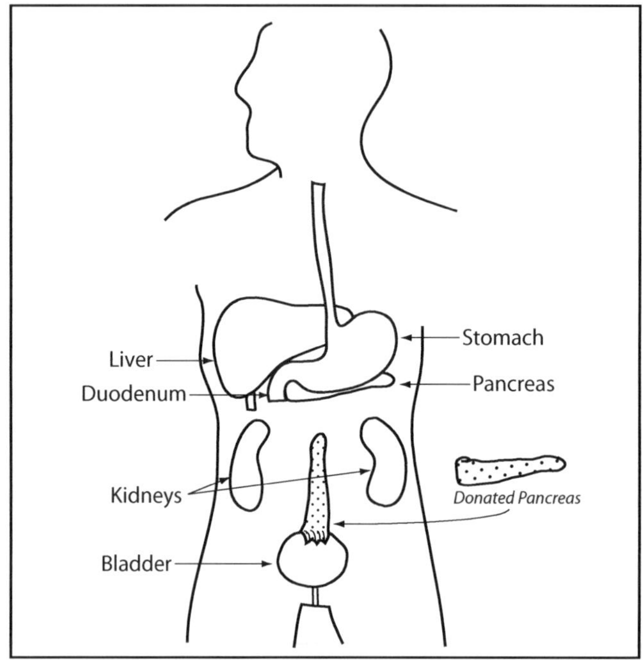

Figure 3: Pancreas Transplantation

abdomen, they would start digesting your insides, causing inflammation and damage. But if they get squirted into your bladder, they get neutralized (or inactivated) in your urine. You get rid of them when you urinate, and so they do not cause problems. One of those enzymes is called amylase.

One of the advantages of attaching the new pancreas to your bladder is that doctors can measure how much amylase is in your urine. If the level of amylase drops, this tells the doctors that the new pancreas is not working as well as it should. This could mean that it is being rejected. Because the new pancreas came from someone else, your own body will recognize it as being "foreign" and will try to reject it. For that reason, you will need to take drugs to suppress your immune system to prevent rejection. Your health care team will measure the amylase level in your urine to check for possible rejection. If your doctors are worried, they might decide to take a small sample of tissue (which is called a biopsy) from the new pancreas to examine it for signs that it is being attacked by your immune system. They can take a biopsy more easily when it is attached to the bladder by inserting their instruments through the urethra (the tube that leads from your bladder to your penis or vagina to allow you to urinate) and into the bladder. They can then push their instruments through the collar of the duodenum and into the transplanted pancreas, where they can snip off a small piece (the biopsy) and pull it all the way back out to be tested.

If the transplant is working well, the islets from the new pancreas begin to measure the glucose level in the blood passing through them and respond to this by making insulin that is released into your bloodstream. This insulin brings your blood glucose down to normal. It is a remarkable process when everything works well. Obviously, there can sometimes be problems. You will certainly need to take immunosuppressive drugs for the rest of your life, and those can have side effects and require regular blood tests and regular checkups. Sometimes the pancreas does not stay as healthy as we would like and does not produce enough insulin to completely cure the person's diabetes.

Who should get a pancreas transplant?

There is a major supply problem for many organ transplantation programs, including pancreas transplant. The number of organ donors who die under circumstances where their pancreas can be removed safely is much fewer than the number of people with diabetes who would like to get a pancreas transplant. For that reason, the transplant teams need to be selective.

Kidney transplantation is a very successful operation for people with diabetes who have severe kidney failure. Most pancreas transplants are done on people who have had diabetes for many years, have kidney failure, and are going to get a kidney transplant to treat that. If there is a pancreas available from the same donor, then a combined kidney plus pancreas transplant can be done. Several hundreds of kidney and pancreas transplants are done in the United States and elsewhere around the world every year.

Several thousand people have had successful pancreas transplants. The chance of having normal blood glucose levels, off insulin, one year after transplant, is about 95 percent if pancreas and kidney transplants are done at the same time. It is about 75 percent if the pancreas transplant is done on its own or is done after the kidney transplant. Part of the increased success of pancreas transplantation when it is done along with a kidney transplant is because it is easier to detect early rejection of the kidney, and so treatment can be changed earlier to protect both the transplanted kidney and pancreas. Most people who get a pancreas transplant have had severe type 1 diabetes for many years. Because it involves major surgery and requires that people take powerful immunosuppressive drugs for the rest of their lives, it is not recommended for children and young adults with recently diagnosed diabetes.

What is the difference between a pancreas transplant and an islet cell transplant?

If you have diabetes, most of your pancreas (99 percent or so) is working properly, producing several pints of digestive juices and enzymes that are pumped into your guts to help you digest your food. The only parts of your pancreas that are not working are the Islets of Langerhans that used to make insulin. So instead of getting a whole pancreas transplanted, an alternative approach is to take the donor pancreas (from an organ donor who recently died) and recover as many healthy islets from it as possible.

A healthy adult pancreas will have between one and two million islets in it. Even with the best techniques, it is usually only possible to recover a few hundred thousand islets or less from the donor pancreas. Those islets are then suspended in a solution of nutrients ready to be injected into the diabetic person who is to get the islet transplant. You might think that those islets are transplanted back into your own pancreas, but that is not technically possible. Instead, they are injected into a large vein (called the portal vein) that takes nutrients from your guts to your liver. The donated islets float down the portal vein and spread out inside your liver, where they get stuck. A new blood supply grows into the islets so that they stay healthy and start measuring your blood glucose and producing insulin in response.

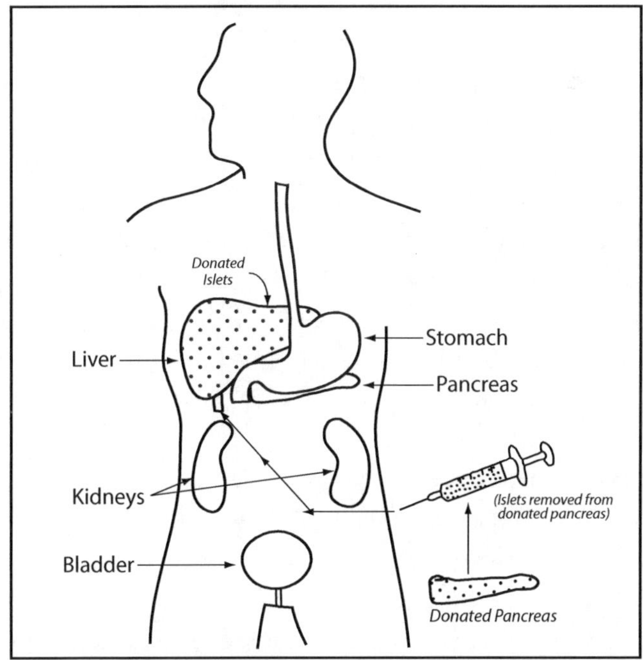

Figure 4: Islet Cell Transplantation

Because the new islets came from someone else, your own body will recognize them as being "foreign" and will try to reject them. For that reason, you will need to take drugs to suppress your immune system to prevent rejection. Some of these drugs actually cause your body to be more resistant to insulin, and others make it hard for the new islets to produce as much insulin as they should. In addition, it is only possible to recover a limited number of islets from the donor pancreas.

For all these reasons, if you get an islet cell transplant, you may need to receive islets from more than a single donor in order to have enough new islets to make enough insulin to cure your diabetes. Sometimes you may not be cured completely but may need to continue taking some insulin shots in addition to the insulin that the islets make.

Who should get an islet cell transplant?

Although there have been significant advances in techniques used with islet cell transplantation in recent years, it is still not a standard form of treatment. Even in centers of excellence where research to improve the treatment is going on all the time, the long term success rate with islet cell transplantation is poor. Only a few hundred people have been given islet cell transplants. On average, they are able to have normal blood glucose levels off insulin for about fifteen months. Only about 10 percent remained cured at five years after the islet cell transplant. For these reasons, islet cell transplants should only be done in centers where research is being done and where the possible risks and benefits are made very clear.

What are stem cells?

You hear a lot about stem cells in the news these days. When a tiny embryo is growing, most of the cells are primitive stem cells. These are cells that can keep dividing and growing but where each cell has not yet determined what type of cell it will grow into. A flippant way to put it is that these young cells haven't decided what they will be when they grow up. Stem cells also have very few protein markers on their surface, so your immune system is less likely to recognize them as being "foreign." So stem cells are less likely to be attacked by your immune system and rejected.

Stem cells can be grown in the laboratory and will keep dividing so that we can end up with large quantities of them. The hope is that once scientists have grown large numbers of stem cells in a laboratory, they may find a way to treat the stem cells in some way to make them turn into a particular type of cell (like a muscle cell or a nerve cell or an insulin-producing cell). So far scientists have not been very successful at doing this, but it is an area of research that holds tremendous promise.

Will stem cells cure diabetes?

One of the reasons why stem cell research is such a hot topic these days is because of the potential it would have to cure illnesses like diabetes. Imagine if scientists could grow unlimited numbers of stem cells in a laboratory and could then stimulate them to turn into insulin-producing cells that could be transplanted into someone with diabetes. We would no longer have a supply problem. And if those stem cells that were making insulin did not have any markers on them telling your body to reject them as being "foreign," then you would not need to take immunosuppressive drugs. Unfortunately, none of those things is possible right now. No one has had diabetes cured by stem cells today. However, you can see that the possibilities are extremely exciting.

What is an artificial pancreas?

An artificial pancreas is a combination of two machines: a continuous glucose monitor and an insulin pump. Two things need to occur for your blood glucose to stay normal without you having to think about it. First, you need a device that will monitor the glucose level in your body every few minutes, twenty-four hours a day, without you having to remember to stick your finger. Second, that glucose information has to be sent to an insulin pump that automatically adjusts the amount of insulin you are getting, in order to keep your glucose in the normal range.

How close are we to having those two things available? For many years we have had insulin pumps that can respond to a continuous glucose monitor. Many pumps already have the kind of infrared (like a television remote) or Bluetooth technology so that they can receive signals from another nearby device. Most insulin pumps deliver insulin through a tiny, soft subcutaneous tube that puts insulin into the fatty tissue under your skin (just like when you give yourself a shot). Researchers have also implanted insulin pumps right inside a person's abdomen so that the insulin can be delivered inside the abdominal cavity. There are technical difficulties with this, but it certainly can be done. Whether the insulin pump is worn externally on your pants' belt or is implanted inside your abdomen, it would still be able to respond to a blood glucose monitor and alter the rate of insulin delivery based on the result.

The problem has been getting a continuous glucose monitor that is reliable. In recent years, there has been great progress. One device is placed on the surface of your skin and stimulates sweat to be pulled through your pores into the device by passing an electric charge across the skin. Since the glucose level in sweat is very close to the glucose level in your blood, this works quite well. There have been technical problems with this device, however. Some people find that it stings to have the electrical stimulation. When I tried it, I thought it felt a bit like a mosquito bite, but I got used to it in a few hours. Another approach is to insert a needle under the skin that measures the glucose level in the interstitial fluid (which is a bit like sweat and, again, gives very similar glucose levels to your blood).

Two companies have got Federal Drug Administration (FDA) approval for their devices so far. You can get more information at www.dexcom.com and www.medtronic.com. At the present time, the glucose sensor part of these continuous blood glucose monitors (the part that is inserted under your skin and measures the blood glucose) needs to be changed to a new location every three to seven days. The idea of connecting the glucose monitor to an insulin pump to make an artificial pancreas is being tested on a research basis but is not available for widespread use yet. I think this is a very promising area of research. I expect to see trials of an insulin pump connected to a continuous glucose monitor in the next couple of years.

Would an artificial pancreas cure diabetes?

If the technical problems can be solved, I am confident that an artificial pancreas would cure diabetes. Let's say you have an insulin pump that is trickling a steady amount of insulin into your body. You have a meal, and your blood glucose begins to go up quickly over the next thirty minutes. Within the first few minutes, the continuous glucose monitor notices that the glucose level is going up. It sends a signal to the insulin pump to start pushing more insulin into your body to bring the blood glucose back down again. As the glucose level falls back toward normal, the continuous glucose monitor notices this trend and tells the insulin pump to back off and give you less insulin. If all of those things happened without you even having to think about it, this would feel very much like a cure for your diabetes.

I think it is most likely that the first versions of an artificial pancreas will be worn on the outside of the body rather than being implanted inside. You should stay tuned for new developments. A good resource for new developments like this is the Juvenile Diabetes Research Foundation (www.jdrf.org).

Does gastric bypass surgery cure type 2 diabetes?

If you have type 2 diabetes and are significantly overweight (with a BMI of over 40kg/m2) and have tried everything you can to change your lifestyle but without success, then gastric bypass surgery is something you should talk to your doctor about as a possibility. It is certainly not for everyone. It is major surgery, and there can be side effects and problems after the surgery is done. For some people, however, it can appear to "cure" their diabetes.

Let's say your own pancreas is working as hard as it can to push out more insulin but because your body is so resistant to the effects of insulin, your blood glucose goes up, and you have type 2 diabetes. If gastric bypass surgery is successful and you lose eighty to a hundred pounds and keep it off, that results in such a dramatic reduction in insulin resistance that the amount of insulin your body makes is now enough to keep your blood glucose completely normal. It can be very dramatic. I have had several patients go through this and come off all of their insulin and pills for diabetes and still have a normal blood glucose.

I hesitate to call it a real "cure" for a couple of reasons. First, you still have to be very careful not to overeat. Having the gastric bypass surgery makes that easier because you feel less hungry, but you can't forget about your eating the way someone without diabetes can. Another problem you will have is that, over time, the amount of insulin that your pancreas makes will continue to fall, and so your diabetes may come back. Even though the results of gastric bypass surgery can sometimes be dramatic in "curing" someone's diabetes, I still tell them that they have really mild and well-controlled diabetes. They should still come in for regular checkups so that they will know if their diabetes comes back later in life.

Part Two: Staying Healthy Longer

Chapter 6

REDUCING CARDIOVASCULAR RISK

- Why are heart attacks and strokes more likely if you have diabetes?
- Why is smoking so much worse for you if you have diabetes?
- What is the easiest way to quit smoking?
- Why is cholesterol bad for you?
- Where does cholesterol come from?
- What is a normal cholesterol level?
- Can you lower your cholesterol with lifestyle changes?
- What drugs can lower your cholesterol?
- Why should I be on a statin drug if my cholesterol is normal?
- What is a normal triglyceride level?
- When should a high triglyceride level be treated?
- What is a normal blood pressure for someone with diabetes?
- What can I do to lower my blood pressure without taking drugs?
- What are the best drugs to lower blood pressure?
- Why should I be on an ACE-inhibitor blood pressure drug if my blood pressure is normal?
- What should I do if I get a persistent cough on an ACE-inhibitor?
- Why should I take aspirin if I have no aches and pains?
- What is the best diet to prevent heart disease?

Why are heart attacks and strokes more likely if you have diabetes?

We don't know all the reasons why, but it is a fact. On average a man with diabetes is twice as likely to have a heart attack or stroke as a non-diabetic man of the same age. Non-diabetic women are less likely to have heart attacks and strokes than non-diabetic men of the same age, but when women get diabetes, they lose that advantage. So women with diabetes are about four times more likely to have a heart attack or a stroke than non-diabetic women of the same age.

Over years a high blood glucose damages the inside of blood vessels. People with diabetes often have higher fat (or lipid) levels (cholesterol and triglyceride) in their blood, especially if the diabetes is poorly controlled, and that can lead to fatty deposits building up in the linings of their blood vessels (a process called atherosclerosis). Those fatty deposits can block the arteries. The lining of your arteries also gets stickier so that blood clots can form inside the blood vessels. When a blood vessel gets blocked, then the tissue that was being supplied with blood, oxygen, and nutrients from that blood vessel gets damaged and dies.

So if a blood vessel supplying the heart muscle (a coronary artery) gets blocked, part of the heart muscle dies. This is called a myocardial infarction, or a heart attack. If an artery supplying the brain gets blocked off, this causes a cerebral infarction, or a stroke. The risk of having a heart attack or stroke depends on how long you have had diabetes, how high your blood glucose has been during those years, and how many other risk factors you have (like smoking, high blood pressure, high cholesterol, and kidney damage). The good news is that although, on average, the risks of having a heart attack or stroke are higher for someone with diabetes, there are a lot of things that you can do to lower that risk enormously.

Why is smoking so much worse for you if you have diabetes?

I know this will sound harsh, but I am going to say it anyway. If you have diabetes and you knowingly and willingly continue to smoke, you must have a death wish. I don't mean to minimize how addictive nicotine is or how hard it is to quit, but quitting smoking is the single most important thing, by far, that you can do to improve your future health if you have diabetes and you smoke.

It is not just a little bit bad for your health; smoking and diabetes is a devastating combination. We don't know all of the reasons why, but here are a few facts. People who need insulin to control their diabetes have a harder time keeping their blood glucose levels near normal if they smoke. Smoking changes the circulation under the skin so that there is more day-to-day variation in insulin absorption. This makes the blood glucose levels more unpredictable throughout the day. People with diabetes who smoke are more likely to get nerve damage (neuropathy) and eye damage (retinopathy). Smoking causes an increase in cholesterol and blood glucose levels and dramatically increases the rate at which your kidneys will get damaged. If you smoke more than fifteen cigarettes a day and have diabetes, you are three times more likely to have a heart attack and twice as likely to die in the next few years as someone with diabetes who doesn't smoke. The risk falls steadily after you quit, however. Diabetic patients who smoke and are on kidney dialysis are four times more likely to die in the next five years than diabetic patients on dialysis who don't smoke.

Here is another way to think about it. The prognosis (the chance of bad things happening to you in the future) in the next ten years is worse for someone with a HbA1c (a measure of blood glucose control) of 7.0 percent who smokes than for someone with a HbA1c of over 9.0 percent who does not smoke! Put another way, quitting smoking does more to improve your future health than dropping your HbA1c by over two percentage points. If you have diabetes and you smoke, there is nothing more important that you can do to improve your health than quitting smoking.

What is the easiest way to quit smoking?

There are no easy ways, but there are a lot of myths and excuses that you should avoid. If you think, "There is no point in trying again; I've tried so many times before without success that I might as well just accept my fate," I'd like you to reconsider. The more often you try to quit, the more likely it is that you will succeed. It sometimes takes people several times before they are successful. Here are some things that might help.

If anyone else in your house also smokes, ask them to quit, too. It will be harder for you to quit if you are kept around the smells and associations that come from someone else smoking. It is also nice to get support from someone else who is going through some of the same problems as you are. Some people find that stopping smoking suddenly ("cold turkey") is too hard because of their nicotine craving. There are a variety of nicotine replacement products (gum, patches, nasal sprays, and inhalers) that are available to allow the nicotine dose to be reduced more gradually. Taking an antidepressant drug like bupropion (Wellbutrin, Zyban) for a few months can help control your craving. Another drug called varenicline (Chantix) has also been shown in randomized clinical trials to increase the chances that people stay quit. You can ask your doctor about whether any of these treatments might help you to quit. There are several organizations that will help you to quit, such as Free and Clear, a telephone-based counseling service that has been shown in well-designed research studies to be effective. You can find out more at www.freeclear.com.

Why is cholesterol bad for you?

There is so much talk on television and other media about drugs to lower cholesterol these days that you might imagine cholesterol is poisonous and that any amount of it in your body or in your blood is bad for you. That is not true. Cholesterol is an important substance in your body. You need cholesterol to help build healthy cell walls. Cholesterol is also a building block for many important hormones in your body. The problem is that there are different kinds of cholesterol, and too much of the bad kind can certainly increase your risk of getting fatty deposits stuck in the lining of your arteries. That can lead to blockage of your arteries, which causes heart attacks, strokes, and many other problems.

The simplest distinction that you will hear is that HDL cholesterol (which stands for high-density lipoprotein cholesterol) is the "good" cholesterol whereas LDL cholesterol (which stands for low-density lipoprotein cholesterol) is the "bad" cholesterol. HDL travels around in your blood vessels cleaning them out, whereas LDL travels around in your blood vessels encouraging fat to be deposited in their lining to block them up. Although that is a bit of an oversimplification, it is not a bad way to think about it. The higher your HDL cholesterol and the lower your LDL cholesterol levels are the less likely you are to have heart attacks and strokes.

Where does cholesterol come from?

You can eat cholesterol in your diet. There is a lot of cholesterol in egg yolks and animal fat, for example, so eating a diet high in animal fat can increase your cholesterol level. But most of the cholesterol in your blood you make yourself in the liver and in your bloodstream. How much cholesterol you have in your blood overall and what proportion is HDL and LDL depends a lot on the genes you inherited from your parents. There are certain things you can do to change those proportions, too. Regular exercise will increase the "good" HDL cholesterol, for example.

What is a normal cholesterol level?

The answer to this question keeps changing. An international group of experts meets every few years to re-examine the scientific evidence and come up with recommended levels for different people. The ideal or "normal" level for you depends on how high your risk is for having heart attacks and strokes in the future. Diabetes is one factor that puts you at higher risk. If you smoke or have high blood pressure or if a close relative had heart disease at an early age, then those factors also increase your risk. For people with diabetes, it is ideal if you can keep your total cholesterol less than 200 mg/dL (5.9 mmol/L), your LDL cholesterol below 100 mg/dL (2.6 mmol/L), and your HDL cholesterol above 60 mg/dL (1.6 mmol/L). Even if you can't get to these ideal levels, the lower you can get the LDL and the higher you can get your HDL, the better.

Can you lower your cholesterol with lifestyle changes?

Improving your diet (by eating less fat overall, especially less animal fat, and increasing the amount of high-fiber carbohydrate) can certainly lower your cholesterol level to some extent. If you have been eating a very high-fat diet, then changing to a healthier diet will have a big effect on lowering your cholesterol. Doing thirty minutes or more of moderate exercise every day will help bring down your LDL and increase your HDL. However, no matter how much you exercise or how much you improve your diet, those things may not be enough to bring your cholesterol down to normal levels if you have inherited the genes that make your body produce too much cholesterol. For that, you will need to take cholesterol-lowering drugs as well.

What drugs can lower your cholesterol?

There are several different types (or classes) of drugs that help lower cholesterol. The most important, by far, are the statins. These drugs have revolutionized the treatment of atherosclerosis (the disease that promotes fat deposits building up inside your blood vessels) and have saved many thousands of lives around the world. There are several available, including lovastatin (Mevacor), pravastatin (Pravachol), simvastatin (Zocor), and atorvastatin (Lipitor). They vary in price (both lovastatin and simvastatin are now generic, which makes them cheaper) and in how powerful they are at bringing your cholesterol down, but the beneficial effects apply to all of them.

The statins are particularly good at bringing down LDL cholesterol. Side effects are remarkably rare. Less than one person in a thousand gets some inflammation of the liver that is bad enough that the drug needs to be stopped. Another side effect is aching muscles. This is usually mild and gets better over time, but occasionally, it can be severe and require that the drug is stopped. It usually takes six weeks after starting a statin (or changing the dose) to see the full effects. So if you are started on one of these drugs, you should expect to be asked to come in for a blood test about six weeks afterward to check how much lower your LDL cholesterol is. A blood test to look for inflammation of the liver may also be done at this time.

There are other drugs that can reduce the amount of cholesterol that you absorb from your intestines. These include cholestyramine (Questran) and ezitimibe (Zetia). You may find cholestyramine less pleasant to take than most drugs since it comes as a gritty powder that you mix with water or juice so that it feels as though you are drinking sand. Most people who take cholestyramine need to take several grams of it a day. However, it is a very safe drug and has been shown in well-designed research studies to lower cholesterol and decrease heart attacks and deaths. Ezitimibe is easier to take but is a newer drug, and so we have no results from research studies telling us whether or not it actually decreases your future risk of heart attacks or stroke or death.

High doses of the B vitamin nicotinic acid can also lower LDL cholesterol and raise HDL cholesterol slightly. The side effects of nicotinic acid include flushing of the skin that some people find very unpleasant. It can also make you more resistant to insulin, and so the drug or insulin treatment that you are taking to control your blood glucose may need to be changed when you take nicotinic acid.

Various natural treatments, including fish oil, can lower your cholesterol and reduce your risk of heart disease. You should talk to your doctor about which ones of all these options might be best for you.

Why should I be on a statin drug if my cholesterol is normal?

A very important research study called the Heart Protection Study (HPS), published in the medical journal *The Lancet* in 2002, followed almost four thousand people who had diabetes but did not have heart disease, as far as they knew. Many of them even had normal cholesterol levels. Those who took 40 mg of simvastatin every day had 30 percent fewer heart attacks during the next five years compared to a matched control group who took a placebo (sometimes called a "sugar" pill or "dummy" pill), even when their cholesterol started out normal and didn't go down that much.

This remarkable result suggests that statin drugs may do more than just lower cholesterol. They may have other effects, such as reducing the inflammation inside your blood vessels. It also means that anyone with diabetes who is over the age of forty should consider starting a statin drug. Some people go as far as to suggest that anyone with diabetes at any age should take a statin, but I disagree with that. The benefit of any drug depends on what your overall risk is. If a twenty-year-old athlete with great cholesterol numbers and no family history of heart disease suddenly develops type 1 diabetes, his or her future risk of getting heart disease is still incredibly small. We have no evidence that starting such a person on a statin would be beneficial. Your risk for heart disease changes over time, so it is a good idea to discuss with your doctor what your risk is and whether a statin or other drug would be a good thing for you to take.

What is a normal triglyceride level?

Triglyceride is another type of fat (or lipid) in your blood. The normal level is less than 150 mg/dL (1.7 mmol/L). A high level can be caused by eating a poor diet, by having your diabetes out of control, and by the genes you inherited.

When should a high triglyceride level be treated?

A high triglyceride level increases your risk for heart disease even when your cholesterol is normal, so it is called an "independent risk factor" for heart disease. If your HDL and LDL cholesterol levels are normal but your triglycerides are above 150 mg/dL (1.7 mmol/L), then your doctor may advise you to take treatment to get it below 150 mg/dL to lower your risk of heart disease. In addition to increasing your risk of heart disease, when the triglyceride levels get very high (over 500 mg/dL, or 5.6 mmol/L), it can cause pancreatitis (inflammation of the pancreas), which can cause severe pains in your abdomen and is a very dangerous condition that usually requires emergency admission to a hospital for treatment. The most common drugs to treat high triglyceride levels are gemfibrozil and fenofibrate.

What is a normal blood pressure for someone with diabetes?

You will hear two numbers when someone tells you your blood pressure. The first number is the systolic blood pressure. This is the pressure inside your arteries when your heart contracts to pump out blood. The second number is the diastolic blood pressure, the lower number that tells us the pressure inside your arteries when the heart muscle relaxes before it beats again with a new contraction. Both systolic and diastolic pressure need to stay within a healthy range to reduce your risk of heart attacks, strokes, kidney damage, and a number of other problems. Because people with diabetes are at higher risk for these things than people who don't have diabetes, the target blood pressure is lower.

Blood pressure levels are measured in old fashioned units that tell how tall a column of liquid mercury can be held up. Some blood pressure machines still use a thin glass column of mercury for measuring blood pressure, but most modern machines don't. It is ideal if you can keep the systolic blood pressure below 130 mmHg (or millimeters of mercury) and the diastolic blood pressure below 80 mmHg. Some people find it easier to control their blood pressure with a combination of changing their diet, exercising more, and taking one or more pills. Even if you can't get your blood pressure below 130/80, the closer to that level you keep it, the better.

What can I do to lower my blood pressure without taking drugs?

The same kind of diet that protects against heart disease and is best to treat diabetes will also help keep your blood pressure lower. A healthy diet should be low in fat (especially animal fat) and high in high-fiber carbohydrates (like lentils, beans, and vegetables). Lowering the amount of protein and salt in your diet can also help reduce your blood pressure. Getting regular exercise and doing things to reduce your stress level will also help to lower your blood pressure.

What are the best drugs to lower blood pressure?

There are many types (or classes) of drug to lower blood pressure. One of the oldest, cheapest, but most important, is thiazide diuretics. These are pills that make you urinate more (some people call them "water pills," because they make your body pass more urine). They are often the first drugs to be used to treat blood pressure. They are not the most powerful blood pressure drug, but even if they are not enough on their own, they help make other blood pressure drugs work better.

Another important class of drugs is called ACE-inhibitors (which stands for Angiotensin Converting Enzyme inhibitors). The names of the ACE-inhibitor drugs all end in "-pril." These include captopril, lisinopril, enalapril, and ramipril, among others. Another class is the Beta-blockers that slow down the heart rate. You may need to take two, three, or even more different types of blood pressure drugs in order to keep your blood pressure down.

Why should I be on an ACE-inhibitor blood pressure drug if my blood pressure is normal?

Several well-designed research studies have showed that, even for people with diabetes who have normal blood pressure, taking an ACE-inhibitor is a good thing to do. These drugs slow down the rate at which the kidneys get damaged from diabetes. They also lower the risk of heart attacks and strokes and seem to protect the eyes from diabetic damage. It is not exactly known why this is. Some doctors are so enthusiastic about the protective benefit of ACE-inhibitors that they say all diabetic patients should take them, no matter how young they are and even if they have normal blood pressure and have no evidence of kidney damage. I think that is going too far. Not only are drugs expensive, they all have side effects.

Before taking any drug, you need to be able to answer the question, will taking this drug likely do me more good than harm? If you are a healthy teenager with well-controlled diabetes, normal blood pressure, and no evidence of kidney damage, the benefits are likely to be tiny, and so the risks of side effects outweigh that benefit. We would have to treat thousands of patients like that for ten years or more before any one of them would gain any benefit. During that time, several of them might develop life-threatening (or even fatal) side effects, so the risks outweigh any benefit. You should certainly talk to your doctor about whether an ACE-inhibitor would be a good idea for you.

What should I do if I get a persistent cough on an ACE-inhibitor?

Some people notice that they get a ticklish, dry cough when they first start taking ACE-inhibitor drugs like enalapril or ramipril. Usually this gets better in a few weeks as your body gets used to the new drug. Starting at a low dose and building the dose up slowly helps. Sometimes the cough was due to something else. Most people have a cough for a few days at some point in any year due to getting a head cold or sore throat from a winter virus.

It is rare for the cough from taking an ACE-inhibitor to be severe and persistent enough to make you want to stop taking the drug, but if it is, there are several options. There is another class of drugs that blocks the receptor that the Angiotensin Converting Enzyme acts on. These ACE receptor blocker drugs usually end in "-artan," so you will see names like losartan or candesartan. These drugs seem to have similar good effects to the ACE-inhibitors, although we do not have as much information about them. They do not cause a cough and so are easier to take for people who have trouble taking ACE-inhibitors. The ACE receptor blockers have not been on the market as long as ACE-inhibitors, and we don't have as many long-term research studies with them, but what we know so far is very encouraging. Like the ACE-inhibitors, they help lower the blood pressure and seem to protect the kidneys from damage that causes you to lose protein in your urine.

Why should I take aspirin if I have no aches and pains?

In addition to being a painkiller and a drug that can reduce fever and inflammation, aspirin makes the platelets in your blood less sticky. Platelets are tiny fragments of cells that float around in your blood and help your blood to clot. Although this is a good thing (to protect you when you cut yourself, for example), it can increase your risk of getting a blood clot in one of your arteries, and that can increase your risk of a heart attack or a stroke.

A low dose of aspirin (81 mg) is recommended for many people with diabetes, especially if they are at increased risk for heart disease. I recommend it to most of my diabetic patients who are over the age of forty. Aspirin is an acid and can sometimes irritate your stomach, but if that is a problem, you can find "enteric-coated" tablets of aspirin available over the counter in most drug stores. This means that the aspirin has been wrapped in a thin layer of material that stops the aspirin from irritating your stomach. Once the pill has passed through the stomach, the thin coating dissolves so that the aspirin can be absorbed into your body without causing the stomach problem.

What is the best diet to prevent heart disease?

There are thousands of diet books out on the market. Some of them have catchy titles or gimmicks that may help you stick to them for a while. Most of them offer sensible advice, but a few are not based on any scientific or nutritional principles at all. You really need to read and compare them with common sense and a healthy dose of skepticism.

Over the past thirty years, some things have been found consistently. It turns out that the same diet that helps protect against obesity helps prevent cancer, heart disease, and diabetes, too. We should all eat less fat, especially animal fat. We should replace saturated animal fat with unsaturated fats, especially monounsaturated fats like olive oil. We should eat more fresh fruits and vegetables, especially those that contain fiber (like lentils and beans). Sometimes it is tricky to eat this kind of diet if you have diabetes. Lots of fresh fruits contain a lot of sugar and so can push your blood glucose levels high. Talking to a nutritionist or dietitian can be very helpful to get advice about how to incorporate these into your diet without causing your blood glucose to go up too much.

Chapter 7

Blood Glucose Control

- What is a normal blood glucose level?
- What is "good blood glucose control" for someone with diabetes?
- What is glycosylated hemoglobin (or hemoglobin A1c, HbA1c)?
- How do I compare the average blood glucose levels from my meter to HbA1c?
- What HbA1c level should I be aiming for if I have diabetes?
- Can it be dangerous to push your HbA1c too low if you have type 2 diabetes?
- How high can the blood glucose level get in someone with diabetes?
- What are ketones?
- When should people with diabetes measure their ketones?
- What is diabetic ketoacidosis?

What is a normal blood glucose level?

The blood glucose level in your blood goes up and down all day long, whether you have diabetes or not. It is usually at its most stable and lowest level when you wake up in the morning and before you have eaten anything. The normal range for this fasting blood glucose is between 70 and 100 mg/dL (3.9–5.9 mmol/L). Your blood glucose goes up after you eat food. How high it goes up and how fast it goes up depends on how much you eat and what type of food you eat. Carbohydrate (especially "simple" or refined carbohydrate like sugar, candy, and regular pop) can be absorbed very quickly and will push the blood glucose up quickly and to high levels for a few minutes at least. For someone without diabetes, it is unlikely to ever get above 160 mg/dL (8.9 mmol/L). If it ever gets above 200 mg/dL (11.1 mmol/L), then you should have it checked a second time, because you may have diabetes. The blood glucose level goes up with food, goes down when you exercise, usually goes up when you are stressed, and goes down when you relax. So even if you do not have diabetes, your blood glucose may go up and down between 70 and 160 mg/dL (3.9–8.9 mmol/L) throughout the day.

What is "good blood glucose control" for someone with diabetes?

There are a couple of different ways to think about this. In order to feel that your diabetes is controlled, you should feel well (not tired or thirsty or stressed out) and able to do everything you want in your life without feeling as though you have to think about your diabetes all the time. Your blood glucose should not be swinging so high that you feel thirsty, exhausted, and needing to go to the bathroom all the time. Your blood glucose should not be dropping so low that you feel sweaty, shaky, and at risk of passing out. In other words, your diabetes should not be constantly disrupting your day to day life.

Once you have accomplished that, it is good to think about what your average blood glucose levels are throughout the day.

Let's compare two people with diabetes. They both feel fine and are getting on with their lives without too much hassle from their diabetes. One of them keeps his blood glucose running between 180 and 300 mg/dL (10–16.7 mmol/L). The other keeps her blood glucose running between 80 and 160 mg/dL (4.4–8.9 mmol/L). Even if both of them feel fine in the short term, over years and years, the woman with the lower blood glucose average is likely to stay a lot healthier and have fewer complications and problems from her diabetes. The higher the average blood glucose level stays, the more likely you are to get damage to your eyes, kidneys, nerves, and blood vessels. So really good blood glucose control is when you can keep your average blood glucose levels close to the normal non-diabetic range without letting it go too low or too high and disrupting your day-to-day life.

What is glycosylated hemoglobin (or hemoglobin A1c, HbA1c)?

Hemoglobin is a protein inside all of your red blood cells. It helps carry oxygen to your tissues to keep you healthy. Every day your body makes a few million new red blood cells in your bone marrow. These get pumped round and round your body for the next two to three months. When the red blood cells get old, your body destroys them in your spleen. Since the hemoglobin is floating around amongst the glucose in your blood, a small amount of glucose gets attached to the hemoglobin. Hemoglobin with glucose attached to it is called glycosylated hemoglobin or hemoglobin A1c (HbA1c). Brand new red cells have no glucose attached to them, but the longer they stay in your bloodstream, the more glucose gets attached. The higher the glucose level in your blood, the more HbA1c you form.

We can measure what percentage of your hemoglobin has glucose attached to it. This tells us what the average glucose level was in your blood for the previous ten to twelve weeks. To give you an idea of how to use this information, a non-diabetic person's blood glucose will vary between about 70 and 160 mg/dL (3.9–8.9 mmol/L) throughout the day. Over time about 4 to 6 percent of the person's hemoglobin will get glycosylated. So the normal range for HbA1c is about 4 to 6 percent. Now, imagine the worst possible blood glucose control. If someone let his or her blood glucose average remain at 400 to 600 mg/dL (22–33 mmol/L) for months on end, the HbA1c could rise above 20 percent. I have never seen HbA1c higher than 25 percent, but it can almost get to that level if someone leaves his or her diabetes completely untreated for long enough.

How do I compare the average blood glucose levels from my meter to HbA1c?

Many blood glucose meters will tell you what your average has been in the past fourteen or thirty days. Researchers have developed a table that compares average blood glucose levels to HbA1c:

Average blood glucose mg/dL (mmol/L)	HbA1c percent
80 mg/dL (4.4 mmol/L)	5.0
120 mg/dL (6.7 mmol/L)	6.0
150 mg/dL (8.3 mmol/L)	7.0
180 mg/dL (10.0 mmol/L)	8.0
210 mg/dL (11.6 mmol/L)	9.0
240 mg/dL (13.3 mmol/L)	10.0
270 mg/dL (15.0 mmol/L)	11.0
300 mg/dL (16.7 mmol/L)	12.0
333 mg/dL (18.5 mmol/L)	13.0
360 mg/dL (20.0 mmol/L)	14.0

You might find this table to be helpful. It shows that if you can improve your average by about 30 mg/dL (1.7 mmol/L) and keep it that much lower for at least three months, then your HbA1c will drop by one whole percentage point.

You should be careful when using this table, however. It only works if your blood glucose average reflects all the ups and downs during the day. When researchers came up with the table, they asked people with diabetes to measure their blood glucose seven times per day (before each of the three main meals, one or two hours after those main meals, and once in the middle of the night). If you only measure your blood glucose when you think it will be low, and if you avoid measuring it when you think it will be high, then the average that you get on your blood glucose meter is not a true average of your blood glucose levels throughout the day.

So if your meter says that your average blood glucose level for the past thirty days is 150 mg/dL (8.3 mmol/L), you would expect from the table that your HbA1c will be 7.0 percent. If it comes back over 9.0 percent, this means that there must be a lot of times during the day when you are not testing but when your blood glucose must be quite high.

What HbA1c level should I be aiming for if I have diabetes?

When researchers have followed groups of people for many years and compared how many of them had heart attacks or damage to their eyes, kidneys, or nerves, they found that there was a strong relationship between all of those problems and what the average HbA1c was during that time. Even among people who don't have diabetes, those who have an HbA1c in the lower end of the normal range (4.0–4.9 percent) have less heart disease in the next five to ten years than those who have an HbA1c in the upper end of the normal range (5.0–5.9

percent). The higher the HbA1c, the more likely it is that there will be damage to the eyes, kidneys, and blood vessels, and the faster those problems will progress. I have illustrated this in the figure below:

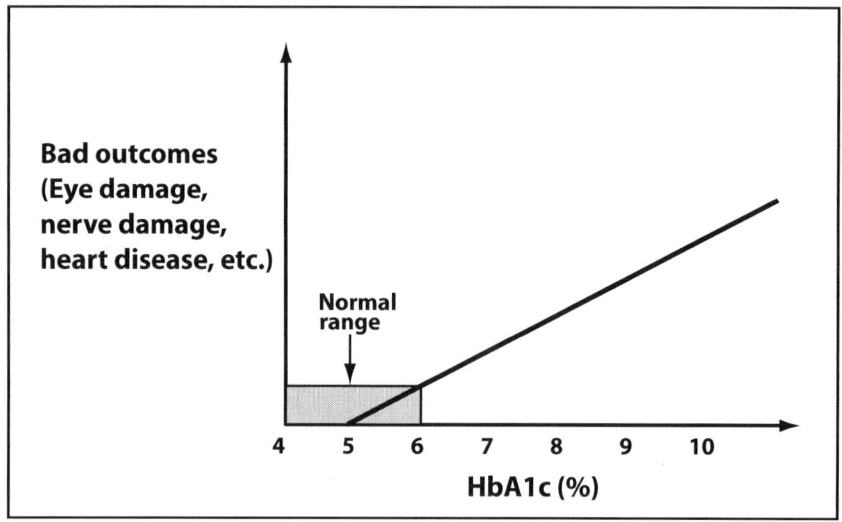

Figure 5: Relationship between HbA1c and Diabetic Complications

Understanding this makes it easier to answer the question in a really practical way. You should try to keep your HbA1c as close to the normal range as possible without ruining your life with the expense and inconvenience and hassle of too many blood glucose tests, too many low blood glucose reactions (which is called hypoglycemia), or too much weight gain or other problems. In other words, you will need to find a balance that works for you. Your doctor and the rest of your health care team should be able to help you pick a target that works for you.

I don't like to see anyone with diabetes going through life with an HbA1c over 9.0 percent, but if the best you can manage without totally disrupting your life is an HbA1c of 9.2 percent, then that is a lot better than having it at 11.2 percent or even higher. But if you could change things to improve your average blood glucose levels by 30 mg/dL (1.7 mmol/L) for at least three months, your HbA1c would come down to 8.2 percent. If you can keep it safely at 7.2 percent, that would be even better. Over years and years, the closer you can keep your HbA1c to the normal non-diabetic range, the healthier you will stay.

Can it be dangerous to push your HbA1c too low if you have type 2 diabetes?

Several studies have tried to answer that question. In one study, over ten thousand people with type 2 diabetes were randomly divided into two groups: one group tried to keep their HbA1c between 7 and 9 percent, and another group tried to keep it as close to 6 percent as possible. After over six years of follow up, the first group had an average HbA1c of 7.5 percent, while the group treated more intensively had an average HbA1c of 6.4 percent. To the surprise of many people, there were more bad outcomes (like heart attacks) in the group with the lower HbA1c. The researchers were unable to say what caused this increase. It is possible that it occurred as a result of side effects of one or more of the drugs used to achieve the lower HbA1c level, but since the same drugs were used in both groups of people, it is not possible to say. Episodes of low blood glucose (hypoglycemia) were more common in the group with the lower HbA1c, but the researchers could not say for sure if this caused the increase in bad outcomes, either. The people who participated in the study were chosen because they were at higher risk of heart disease to begin with, and their average age was over sixty. Until we know more from further research, it may be better to keep the HbA1c between 7 and 8 percent if you are over sixty years of age and if you are at higher than normal risk for heart disease.

How high can the blood glucose level get in someone with diabetes?

When the blood glucose gets above 180 mg/dL (10 mmol/L), your kidneys start to filter glucose out of the blood, and you pass it in your urine. The higher the blood glucose gets, the more your kidneys filter out; so people with very high blood glucose levels start to urinate large quantities of glucose and water in their urine. This is why people get very dehydrated and thirsty when their diabetes is uncontrolled. When you get dehydrated, your blood gets more concentrated, and so the blood glucose level gets higher.

If your kidneys are not able to filter glucose fast enough, then that can cause glucose to build up even higher in your blood. I have seen quite a few teenage patients over the years walk into my office with their blood glucose between 500 and 1000 mg/dL (28–56 mmol/L) and HbA1c values over 20 percent. I have been amazed that they were still able to walk and function! Many people would be so ill with glucose levels that high that they would collapse or pass out and would need to be admitted to the hospital. It is amazing what the human body can sometimes tolerate for short periods of time, but it is very unhealthy for the blood glucose to stay above 200 mg/dL (11.1 mmol/L) for long periods of time.

What are ketones?

If people who do not have diabetes eat fewer calories than their body needs, their pancreas will stop pushing insulin into their blood. With no insulin around, the body's stores of fat begin to break down. When fat breaks down, it produces ketones, a kind of organic solvent like acetone. Ketones smell a bit like nail-polish remover or paint stripper. If you have a sensitive nose, you may be able to detect the fruity smell of acetone on the breath of someone who is dieting.

If you have diabetes and do not have enough insulin in your blood and elsewhere in your body, then you will start to break down fat and produce ketones. This can happen in a matter of a few hours if you forget to take an insulin shot or if you run out of insulin or if your insulin has gone off by being left baking in the sun, for example. It can also happen if you get sick with a cold or the flu or get a urinary or other infection. When you get sick, your body releases a lot of "stress hormones," like cortisol and adrenaline. These make it harder for your insulin to work properly, so even if you are taking your usual dose of insulin, it may not be enough to overcome the effects of these stress hormones. As a result, you begin to break down fat and produce ketones. Those ketones can be detected in your blood and also in your urine. It is easier to measure ketones in the urine, and most drugstores will sell test strips to allow you to test for ketones in your urine. These are sometimes called "ketostix."

When should people with diabetes measure their ketones?

If you are taking insulin, and especially if you have type 1 diabetes, it is a good idea to keep some "ketostix" with you to test for ketones when your blood glucose is high for no obvious reason. There are two main ways for your blood glucose to go over 300 mg/dL (16.7 mmol/L) if you have diabetes. If you eat a large amount of carbohydrate, and don't take enough insulin to cover it, then it is easy for the blood glucose to get over 300 mg/dL. It is unlikely that you will have ketones in your urine under this circumstance. However, if you are coming down with an illness and your insulin is not working properly, then your blood glucose can get high because of your lack of insulin. You need insulin to push glucose out of your blood and into the muscle, fat, liver, and other cells where it is needed.

If your blood glucose is high because your insulin level is too low, you will be spilling a lot of ketones in your urine, because the lack of insulin also makes your body start to break down fat. A high blood glucose that is associated with you spilling ketones in your urine is serious. You should contact your health care team and ask for advice. You may need to drink more fluids to stop becoming dehydrated. You may need to take more insulin than usual. You may need to come in to be examined by a doctor. The presence of ketones in your urine is often an early warning sign that you are getting sick and need extra help and attention.

What is diabetic ketoacidosis?

This dangerous condition is a combination of high blood glucose levels, acidic blood, dehydration, electrolyte imbalance, and excess ketone production. It is a real medical emergency. If your body has too little insulin and this situation goes on for several hours or days, you can become very sick and even die.

You need insulin to help push glucose out of the blood into all the cells that need that glucose for energy. Insulin also helps keep the chemical balance in your body correct. If you have too little insulin, then potassium leaks out of your cells and your body breaks down fat and produces ketones. Some of those ketones are acidic. Your blood glucose level climbs higher and higher; you become dehydrated; you lose potassium and other chemicals in your urine. You produce too much acid in your blood. You become exhausted. Your brain finds it harder and harder to function, and you become drowsy. The chemical imbalance in your blood makes your heart muscle get irritable.

If diabetic ketoacidosis is left untreated, you could pass into a coma and could develop a severe heart rhythm problem and could die. Without prompt treatment, most people with diabetic keto-acidosis will die in a few hours.

Chapter 8

HYPOGLYCEMIA

- What is hypoglycemia?
- What causes hypoglycemia?
- What are the symptoms of hypoglycemia?
- What should I do if I feel hypoglycemic symptoms coming on?
- How many tablets of glucose should I take to treat hypoglycemia?
- What should I take to treat hypoglycemia if I am away from home and don't have glucose tablets with me?
- Do hypoglycemic symptoms occur at the same blood glucose level every time?
- If I feel more comfortable when my glucose levels are higher, why should I risk hypoglycemia?
- Isn't hypoglycemia dangerous?
- Can hypoglycemia cause an epileptic seizure?
- Can hypoglycemia damage your brain cells?
- Can you ever have hypoglycemia without knowing it?
- If I wake up with a headache, does that mean I was hypoglycemic during the night?
- Can people who don't have diabetes get hypoglycemia?
- If I had hypoglycemia and passed out unconscious, would I die?
- What can someone else do to help me if I pass out unconscious from hypoglycemia?
- Am I safe from hypoglycemia if I eat extra food while I exercise?
- Why can't I recognize my hypoglycemia symptoms like I used to?
- Is it safe to drive if I might have hypoglycemia?
- What is a safe blood glucose to go to bed with to avoid hypoglycemia during the night?

What is hypoglycemia?

The medical term for a blood glucose that is too low is hypoglycemia. When the blood glucose level falls below the normal fasting range of 70–100 mg/dL (3.9–5.6 mmol/L), this causes problems. Your brain needs glucose to function properly. Glucose is the only fuel that your brain uses, in fact, so if the glucose level falls too low, your brain quickly does several things to try to push your blood glucose up again. If your blood glucose kept going down, you would pass out into a coma and your brain would have a seizure.

What causes hypoglycemia?

Any combination of too much insulin, too little food, and too much exercise can lead to hypoglycemia. It is rare for people who don't have diabetes to develop hypoglycemia, because when the blood glucose level falls too low, their body can turn off the cells that are making insulin. If you have diabetes and are taking insulin shots, you can't turn that insulin off once it has been injected. And if you have type 2 diabetes and take pills that stimulate your own pancreas to push out insulin, you can't stop that insulin from being pushed out, even when your blood glucose falls too low.

So if you have diabetes, there are several situations that can cause your blood glucose to get too low. If you take too much insulin or too high a dose of an insulin-stimulating pill, you can get hypoglycemia. If you take the correct dose of your insulin or pill but eat too little carbohydrate food or wait too long between taking your insulin and starting to eat, then you can get hypoglycemia. If you take your usual dose of insulin or insulin-stimulating pill and take your usual amount of food but do much more exercise than usual, then that can cause hypoglycemia.

What are the symptoms of hypoglycemia?

When your blood glucose gets too low, your brain "presses the panic button" by telling your adrenal glands to pour out adrenaline (epinephrine) and nor-adrenaline (norepinephrine). These are the same hormones that get released when you get a sudden scare, like when someone jumps out of the bushes to surprise you or when a dog snarls or tries to bite you. Adrenaline and noradrenaline are often called the "fight or flight" hormones. They prepare your body very quickly to either stay where you are and fight the threat or to take flight and run away from the situation. They make your heart start to race. Your body trembles, you start to sweat, you feel anxious, and you look pale. You can feel any or all of those symptoms when your blood glucose gets too low.

If your blood glucose keeps dropping, your brain stops working properly. You may get drowsy and confused. You may slur your speech and seem "spacey." Some people seem to get a personality change and become much more grumpy and bad-tempered than they usually are. If nothing is done to bring your blood glucose back up, you may even pass out into a coma.

In summary the symptoms you get are either due to an "adrenaline rush" or to your brain and nervous system being starved of glucose. Here is a list of the main symptoms of hypoglycemia:

- Sweating
- Trembling
- Shaking
- Feeling hungry
- Feeling anxious
- Having a rapid pounding heart rate
- Tingling and numbness (sometimes around the mouth)
- Change in color (people might notice that you look pale)
- Drowsiness

- Confusion or slurred speech
- Acting "spacey" or appearing to be intoxicated
- Change in personality (often seeming grumpy, argumentative, and unreasonable)

What should I do if I feel hypoglycemic symptoms coming on?

One problem with the symptoms of hypoglycemia is that they could be caused by other things, so you should first check your blood glucose to be sure. This can sometimes be tricky. If you suddenly feel sweaty and anxious and think you are going to pass out, then the desire to cram carbohydrates into your mouth can be so strong that you may not want to take the time to check your blood glucose. You need to use sensible judgment.

If you are sure that your blood glucose is dropping too low, you should take fast-acting carbohydrate as soon as possible. The best thing to take is glucose, which comes in tablets or as a liquid gel. If you feel that you do have time to test your blood glucose before you eat some carbohydrate, this can be very helpful. It lets you know just how low your blood glucose is. You can check it again every ten minutes or so after you take some food so that you can see how quickly you respond.

How many tablets of glucose should I take to treat hypoglycemia?

Glucose tablets usually come in 5-gram sizes. Taking three tablets (about 15 grams of glucose) right away will begin to bring your blood glucose up in just a few minutes. You should follow this with a larger amount of more long-lasting carbohydrate (such as a sandwich, crackers, or a granola bar). It is a good idea to carry a supply of glucose with you wherever you go or to make sure you have some in your purse, clothes, at your desk at work, in your car, or wherever you might need it in a hurry. You should also have more long-lasting carbohydrate and protein snacks available, too, to take once your blood glucose has come up with the glucose tablets. Remember, taking a few glucose tablets may only keep your blood glucose up for a few minutes.

What should I take to treat hypoglycemia if I am away from home and don't have glucose tablets with me?

If you don't have glucose available, then drinking half a can of regular (*not* diet) pop or juice (like apple juice or orange juice) or eating some hard candy (*not* sugar free candy) is a reasonable alternative. Glazed doughnuts and cake frosting also work well. Some of my patients tell me that they look forward to becoming hypoglycemic because it gives them an excuse to eat all the things that are "forbidden" at other times! Again, follow up by eating something more substantial afterward, or else your blood glucose might start dropping again after the small amount of glucose has been used up.

Do hypoglycemic symptoms occur at the same blood glucose level every time?

No, they don't. People vary a lot it in what symptoms they get and what blood glucose level they need to be at to get those symptoms. If you have had high blood glucose averages (let's say over 200 mg/dL, or 11.1 mmol/L) for a long time, you might start feeling hypoglycemic symptoms when your blood glucose falls below 100 mg/dL (5.6 mmol/L). But if your body is more used to lower blood glucose levels and your average blood glucose is 120 mg/dL (6.7 mmol/L), then you may not feel hypoglycemic symptoms until your blood glucose is less than 60 mg/dL (3.3 mmol/L) or even lower.

Symptoms sometimes come on at higher levels if your blood glucose is dropping fast. If your blood glucose is dropping very slowly, it can sometimes get a lot lower before you realize you are low and symptoms start. If you are wide awake and alert, you will tend to notice your hypoglycemic symptoms at higher blood glucose levels than you will if you are sleepy or distracted. People who drink coffee or other caffeinated products often notice their hypoglycemic symptoms at higher blood glucose levels.

If I feel more comfortable when my glucose levels are higher, why should I risk hypoglycemia?

The way you feel when your blood glucose is too low can be very scary and uncomfortable. I totally understand why you might want to avoid it at all costs. But over years, there is much more danger from high blood glucose levels damaging your body than from low blood glucose. If you can learn to recognize when your blood glucose is dropping low and learn to treat it quickly and effectively without getting too stressed out about it, you are more likely to be able to keep your average blood glucose level closer to normal. People who keep their blood glucose over 200 mg/dL (11.1 mmol/L) all the time may feel happy that they don't ever get hypoglycemic symptoms, but after a few years of keeping the blood glucose so high, they are much more likely to get problems from damage to their eyes, kidneys, nerves, and blood vessels.

Isn't hypoglycemia dangerous?

Yes, hypoglycemia can be dangerous. If you became drowsy or confused or passed out from hypoglycemia while you were driving a car or using dangerous equipment like a chain saw, you could certainly injure or kill yourself or others. It is important to learn which situations can make hypoglycemia likely, learn to recognize the early warning symptoms, have glucose and other food available at all times to treat hypoglycemia. It is also good to let people you are close to know that you have diabetes and teach them how they can help you if your blood glucose drops too low.

Can hypoglycemia cause an epileptic seizure?

Yes, it can. If the brain gets starved of glucose for long enough, it will get irritable and can "fire off" in an uncoordinated way that results in a seizure. Although it is rarely done nowadays, doctors used to give "insulin shock therapy" to treat people with severe depression. They would inject a big enough dose of insulin into patients to push their blood glucose so low that they would have a seizure. This did, in fact, often improve their symptoms of depression, but it is considered too dangerous to be used anymore.

Can hypoglycemia damage your brain cells?

If your blood glucose stayed really low for several hours, it could damage your brain cells. If you have had diabetes for many years and if your blood glucose has gone really low several times, it is possible that some of your brain cells could be damaged. Research studies have tested people with diabetes to see how fast their reflexes are or how quickly they can do math or shape identification problems. When compared with people of the same age who do not have diabetes, the people with diabetes are very slightly worse at some of those tests. However, the differences are usually so tiny that you could hardly tell any difference at all in day-to-day life. I have friends and colleagues who have had diabetes for forty years or more and are still incredibly bright and sharp, doing complicated and demanding jobs. Over many years, there is far more risk to your overall health from keeping your blood glucose too high than from episodes of hypoglycemia.

Can you ever have hypoglycemia without knowing it?

Yes, you can. If you have diabetes and take insulin, it is perfectly possible for your blood glucose to drop into the hypoglycemic range for several hours during the night while you are asleep. Even if you test your blood glucose when you wake up and it is high, it is still quite possible that you had hypoglycemia during the night. If you often wake up feeling tired or have a headache or find that your nightclothes are wet from sweat, these may be signs that you had a really low blood glucose during the night.

It is also quite common for you to have a low blood glucose level sometime when you are tired or are distracted and not realize that you are low. Sometimes a close friend or family member will notice it before you do. They may notice that you look pale or sweaty or that you are acting oddly. If someone you know and trust tells you that they think your blood glucose is low, it is a good idea to check it, even if you feel fine.

If I wake up with a headache, does that mean I was hypoglycemic during the night?

If you wake up with a headache, it might mean that your blood glucose was low during the night, but there are other causes of early morning headache. If you also feel tired and sweaty, or if your nightclothes are wet, then that makes it more likely that your headache was caused by hypoglycemia during the night. If this happens more than once, then it is a good idea to set your alarm for the middle of the night a few times and check how low your blood glucose is while you are sleeping. If your overnight blood glucose levels are less than 80 mg/dL (4.4 mmol/L), then you should see your doctor to get help making adjustments to your diabetes treatment to avoid hypoglycemia during the night. But if your blood glucose levels are always over 80 mg/dL during the night and you are still waking up with headaches, then you should ask your doctor if you need to be tested for other causes of headache.

Can people who don't have diabetes get hypoglycemia?

Yes, they can, but it is much rarer than most people think. "Hypoglycemia" is often over-diagnosed in people who don't have diabetes. Here's how it can happen. People get symptoms where they feel weak, sweaty, dizzy, hungry, or peculiar in some way, in between meals. They may think they have hypoglycemia. They go to a doctor who gives them an oral glucose tolerance test (OGTT). The doctor may even tell them that this test confirms that they have hypoglycemia. Truthfully, this is a very bad way to try to make the diagnosis of hypoglycemia.

When you get an oral glucose tolerance test, you are told to eat and drink nothing except plain water for over ten hours before the test starts. You are then given a large amount of sugary liquid to drink very quickly. You then get your blood glucose tested every half hour for several hours, without being allowed to eat anything. It is quite possible and normal for people without diabetes to respond to that test by having their blood glucose drop down below 60 mg/dL (3.3 mmol/L) three or four hours after the glucose drink. They may well feel awful by that point, too. This does *not* mean that they have a diagnosis of hypoglycemia or that they need to change their diet and eat lots of small meals containing carbohydrate and protein.

If people without diabetes think that they may be having hypoglycemic symptoms from time to time they should get blood tests done at the time when they get their funny symptoms. Those tests should measure the level of glucose and insulin and C-peptide in their blood. If either the insulin or C-peptide levels (or both) are inappropriate for the blood glucose level, then further testing is worthwhile. However, many times when those tests are done, they confirm that the blood glucose is not low and that the insulin and C-peptide levels are normal, so that the person's "hypoglycemic symptoms" are actually due to something else.

If I had hypoglycemia and passed out unconscious, would I die?

This is a very real concern that you may have, but the truth is, it is incredibly rare for hypoglycemia to cause someone to die, even if they pass out and are unconscious for a few hours. Obviously if you pass out unconscious from hypoglycemia while you are driving or operating dangerous equipment, you could be killed. But if you became unconscious from hypoglycemia during the night while you were sleeping, you would most likely just wake up a few hours later. Here's why.

Let's say you took too big of a dose of insulin before you went to bed (or you had too little food or did too much exercise during the evening before you went to bed), and you became hypoglycemic while you were asleep and became unconscious. After a few hours, the insulin shot would wear off and the level of insulin in your blood would fall. In addition, your body would start pouring out adrenaline, noradrenaline, and other hormones like glucagon, cortisol, and growth hormone. All of those hormones can force your liver to release glucose into the bloodstream to bring your blood glucose back up. We each carry about 300 grams of glucose stored in our liver in the form of a compound called glycogen. That is the equivalent of having twenty slices of bread stored in your liver. When your insulin level falls and when those other hormone levels rise, your liver turns that glycogen into glucose, and you wake up.

I don't mean to minimize the seriousness of hypoglycemia. It is not good to pass out unconscious from it. If your blood glucose got low enough, you could have an epileptic seizure and choke on your tongue or on vomit, if you threw up. It is a good thing to avoid really low blood glucose levels during the night, and if someone ever finds you unconscious from hypoglycemia, I would want them to call 9–1-1 and to do other things to treat you to bring your glucose up, if they know how to. But I do want you to know that the vast majority of people who pass out unconscious from hypoglycemia simply wake up a few hours later. They will likely feel exhausted from the experience and will definitely want to learn how to avoid it in future.

What can someone else do to help me if I pass out unconscious from hypoglycemia?

They should certainly try to rouse you and see if you are able to eat or drink some glucose or a regular pop or juice. If you are unconscious and cannot be roused, they should call 9–1-1. There are other things that someone else can do if they have been shown how. If the liquid gel glucose paste is smeared inside your lips or under your tongue, you may absorb enough of it to bring your blood glucose level up so that you come to and can then drink some more glucose and eat something.

A close friend or relative may also be taught to give you an injection of glucagon. Glucagon is one of the hormones that your body pushes out in response to a low blood glucose. It is available as a kit so that someone can inject it into you if you are unconscious. A glucagon kit usually contains a small container of glucagon powder and a syringe with a needle and sterile water in it. The glucagon is kept as a powder to make it last longer. If it was already mixed up in solution, it would "go off" quicker. Your friends or relatives will be taught to inject the liquid into the bottle of powder and shake it up to dissolve the glucagon. They would then draw it back up into the syringe and inject it under your skin. Some people worry that there might be bubbles in the syringe and that those bubbles might cause harm to you, but that is extremely unlikely. The glucagon injection should be given into your subcutaneous fat or muscle. They will be taught how to do this. Usually injecting glucagon into your buttock or leg or abdomen works very well. You will probably come to within five minutes. You may well feel nauseous and have a headache, but you can usually understand what is going on by then and drink some glucose and eat some food to keep your blood glucose up. If no one has glucose paste or glucagon to treat you, then the paramedics who arrive in response to the 9–1-1 call will give you an injection of glucose directly into one of your veins, and that will bring you round.

Am I safe from hypoglycemia if I eat extra food while I exercise?

It is certainly a good idea to check your blood glucose frequently before, during, and after exercise and to take extra food. But if you have done a prolonged amount of vigorous exercise (like several hours of playing basketball or cycling, for example), then there is a risk that your blood glucose will continue to fall for several hours afterward, so you might have severe hypoglycemia many hours later. Here's why.

I mentioned that we all keep a store of glucose in our liver in the form of a substance called glycogen. We also have a store of glycogen in our muscles. When you begin to exercise, your muscles burn up all of the glycogen inside them in the first half hour or so. The muscles then send out signals to your liver to release glucose from the glycogen that is stored there. You may also eat extra carbohydrate during your exercise so that your muscles keep having a supply of glucose to burn. When you finish your exercise, even if your blood glucose is normal at that time, your muscles will continue to pull glucose out of your blood for several more hours in order to build up their store of glycogen again. For that reason, it is a good idea to have an extra big snack after a vigorous workout, especially one that contains a lot of slowly released carbohydrate, to keep your glucose up for the next several hours. A peanut butter and jelly sandwich works well for some people. There are also special bars you can buy that contain uncooked cornstarch. They work well to give you sustained amounts of glucose for several hours.

Why can't I recognize my hypoglycemia symptoms like I used to?

It used to be thought that once you had diabetes for many years, you simply lost the ability to recognize hypoglycemia symptoms anymore. Many doctors think this, too, and tell their patients that nothing can be done about it. This is a myth! It is usually quite easy to regain your ability to recognize low blood glucose levels.

It may help you to understand why you lost the ability to recognize your low blood glucose levels in the first place. Any time your blood glucose falls below normal, your body makes an adjustment so that for the next two to three days it will be less able to recognize another episode of hypoglycemia. In fact, if you have another hypoglycemic episode in the next couple of days, your body will not respond as vigorously to bring your blood glucose back up. The amounts of adrenaline and the other hormones that it pushes out to help bring your blood glucose up will be less after the second episode. And if you keep having frequent episodes of hypoglycemia, the situation gets worse and worse, until you feel as if you don't recognize them and don't respond to them. It can be very scary. This can happen if you are having low blood glucose levels for several hours every night without knowing it. In a matter of days, your body will stop reacting properly to hypoglycemia even when it happens during the day.

The way to treat this is to talk to your doctor about changing some of the things you are doing for your diabetes. You may need to take a lower dose of insulin or change the type of insulin you are taking or when you are taking it. You might need to change what and when you eat or what kind of exercise you do and when you do it. If you can make adjustments so that, for at least a week, your blood glucose never drops below 100 mg/dL (5.6 mmol/L), then your body's ability to recognize hypoglycemia and respond to it should get much better again.

Is it safe to drive if I might have hypoglycemia?

That is a judgment call you need to make. Having a hypoglycemic episode while you are driving is one of the most dangerous situations for someone with diabetes. You could pass out, crash your car, and kill yourself and others. You should certainly wear a MedicAlert bracelet (www.medicalert.com) so that if you did pass out or crash, the medics would know that you have diabetes. I know several people with diabetes who have been pulled over by the police for driving erratically and who were accused of being drunk or under the influence of other drugs when, in fact, they were hypoglycemic. Wearing something that identifies you as having diabetes can help you in that situation.

For most people with diabetes, driving is quite safe. You need to be tuned in to what your earliest symptoms of hypoglycemia usually are. People vary in what symptoms they feel first. Do you usually notice you are sweating or trembling or your heart races or you feel tired or hungry? You should check your blood glucose before you set out to drive. You should be aware of whether your blood glucose is likely to be going up or down in the next hour. This will depend on when you took your pills or insulin, when you last ate, what you ate, and whether you have recently exercised. You should keep a supply of glucose tablets or glucose paste or fruit juice near at hand, along with other snacks of carbohydrate and protein that will help keep your blood glucose up longer. If you are going on a journey of longer than an hour, you should stop and recheck your blood glucose once or twice. You should check your blood glucose when you arrive.

You may not need to do this much blood glucose checking for every journey, but it is a good idea to do it for journeys of a variety of lengths and at different times of the day to get a sense of what typically happens to your blood glucose in different situations. If you have had a recent severe hypoglycemic episode requiring the help of someone else, or if you have lost the ability to tell when your hypoglycemia is coming on, you should seriously consider NOT driving until you have seen your doctor to get the situation addressed. If you are involved in an accident due to hypoglycemia, you may have your license suspended for several months until a doctor tells your licensing agency that you are safe to drive again.

What is a safe blood glucose to go to bed with to avoid hypoglycemia during the night?

This really depends on what type of treatment you are taking for your diabetes. If you are only taking metformin for your diabetes, then it is very unlikely that your blood glucose will go too low during the night. But if you take a drug that forces your pancreas to push out extra insulin, or if you are taking shots of insulin, you should not go to bed with a blood glucose under 100 mg/dL (5.6 mmol/L). How low your blood glucose drops during the night depends on the type of insulin you are taking, how much you have eaten during the evening, and how much exercise you have had. I'm afraid there is no "magic number" I can give you that says, "If you are above this blood glucose level, you will be safe to go to sleep."

Chapter 9

PREVENTING EYE DAMAGE

- How does a high blood glucose cause damage to the eyes?
- If I have diabetes, does that mean I will go blind one day?
- Why does my vision get worse when my blood glucose levels change?
- Why should I get my eyes checked regularly when my eyesight is fine?
- How often do I really need to get my eyes checked?
- What are doctors looking for when they check your eyes?
- If another family member has diabetic eye damage, does that mean I am at more risk of getting it, too?
- What is laser therapy?
- What is a vitrectomy?
- If I have diabetic retinopathy, should I stop taking aspirin?
- Apart from getting regular eye exams, what else can I do to prevent eye damage?

How does a high blood glucose cause damage to the eyes?

We don't know all of the ways that high blood glucose levels can damage the eyes. The eye is a globe. There is a hard clear lens at the front of the eye that focuses images on the back part of the eye (which is called the retina). The middle part of the globe is filled with a clear liquid called the vitreous. There are protein membranes lining lots of tiny blood vessels in the retina (the layer that contains all of the nerve cells that allow you to detect light and color and send the information to your brain). It is possible that glucose gets attached to those proteins to damage and weaken them. They then begin to leak fat or blood out of the vessels into the retina nearby. The weaker linings of the blood vessels begin to bulge out (like a blowout on a rubber bicycle tire). These "blowouts" are called aneurysms. Your body tries to repair these weakened areas by making more lining cells. These new cells fill up the aneurysm but can sometimes end up blocking the blood vessel altogether. The part of your retina that is beyond the blockage then gets starved of oxygen and nutrients, and so the retina stops working properly in that area of your eye.

If this condition progresses, your body responds by growing new blood vessels inside your eye. These often grow quickly and in an uncoordinated way, creating a tangled mass of fragile new blood vessels. The blood vessels may rupture, causing major bleeding within your eye. Even if they do not bleed, these new blood vessels tend to develop scar tissue around them. When the scars contract, they can distort the lining of your eye and can grow over the retina so that your vision becomes severely impaired.

If I have diabetes, does that mean I will go blind one day?

Not at all. Most people with diabetes keep good vision through their entire life. There are things you can do to make it much less likely that you will get damage to your eyes. Keeping good blood glucose control (with your HbA1c under 7.0 percent, if possible), keeping your blood pressure well controlled (below 130/80), and not smoking will all reduce your risk of getting eye damage in the future. Getting regular eye examinations can detect problems years before they would ever affect your vision. There are treatments that can prevent deterioration of your vision.

Why does my vision get worse when my blood glucose levels change?

When your blood glucose levels are high, your body holds on to more water in order to keep the high levels of glucose dissolved in your blood and other tissues. Your eyeball swells up with this extra water. The vitreous part of your eye can adapt and swell up quite quickly, but the lens, which is a much harder substance, takes much longer to swell up with the extra fluid. This means that there are times when your lens is the wrong size for the rest of your eyeball, and so your vision will be blurred. This is not a dangerous or permanent problem, but it can be really annoying. When you improve your blood glucose control and bring your average glucose levels down, then your eyeball and lens start to shrink back to their normal size. Once again the vitreous shrinks faster than the lens, and so for several days or weeks, your vision will be blurred again.

The most important thing to remember is that this is not a sign of serious eye damage but is something that will get better once your lens and vitreous are back to their correct size. Make sure that you don't go and get a new prescription for eyeglasses or contact lenses during this time, or you will waste money. Once your eyes have adjusted back to their normal size, your new glasses won't work anymore.

Why should I get my eyes checked regularly when my eyesight is fine?

In the early stages of eye damage from diabetes (which is called diabetic retinopathy), you won't have any symptoms at all. Your vision will be just fine. The only way to know what is happening inside your eyes at this stage is to have an eye doctor look inside through a special instrument (called an ophthalmoscope) or to take a photograph of the back of your eye using a special retinal camera. Usually this is done after putting drops in your eyes to dilate your pupils. Some retinal cameras can take good photographs through undilated pupils, but for a routine eye examination, you should expect to get your eyes dilated. It usually takes many years for diabetic retinopathy to progress to the point where it will affect your vision. By checking regularly, treatment can be started well ahead of time to preserve your vision and protect your eyes.

How often do I really need to get my eyes checked?

If you have type 2 diabetes, you should get a dilated eye examination as soon as you have been diagnosed. It is possible that your blood glucose has been above normal for several years and you did not know. That could mean that you already have some damage at the back of your eyes.

If you have type 1 diabetes, it is not necessary to get a dilated eye examination until you have had diabetes for five years. If your first dilated eye examination is perfectly normal, you only need to get the test repeated every two years. Some people prefer to get their eyes examined every year. This is especially important if you have poor blood glucose control or if you have high blood pressure or if you smoke. If your eye doctor tells you that you have developed some damage to the back of your eye from diabetes, then you will be asked to have the dilated eye examination more often (at least once a year).

What are doctors looking for when they check your eyes?

An eye doctor will test the pressure in your eyes to make sure it is not too high (a condition called glaucoma). He or she will also check to see if the lens inside your eye is clear or is turning opaque in places (causing a cataract). When an eye doctor looks in the back of your eye, he or she can see if the tiny blood vessels in your retina are healthy or whether they have bulges on them (aneurysms) or are leaking fat or blood out of them. The eye doctor will also check to see if there is too much fluid around the macula (which is the part of your retina you use when you are focusing on details). He or she will also look for fragile new blood vessels or scar tissue growing inside your eye.

If another family member has diabetic eye damage, does that mean I am at more risk of getting it, too?

Yes, it does. People vary in how long their blood vessels can tolerate high blood glucose levels, and the genes you inherited play a part. Some families have several members with diabetes, but none of them seem to get eye problems, even after several decades of diabetes. You could say that those families have genes that make the linings of their blood vessels tough and resistant to damage from high blood glucose. For other families, eye problems seem to start after only a few years. Obviously, two different family members may have different levels of interest in their diabetes and different levels of glucose control. If one brother had an HbA1c of over 9.0 percent for years and his sister kept her HbA1c below 7.0 percent, I would expect her to have fewer eye problems than her brother. But even when we take these differences into account, there are family similarities about how early eye damage can start. So if you have someone in your family who already has diabetes and has eye damage, make sure that you get tested regularly.

What is laser therapy?

If an eye doctor has been following you and the amount of retinopathy is progressing and getting worse every year, then the eye doctor might suggest that you get laser therapy. What they do is to fire a tiny laser beam very carefully and precisely onto the back of your eye (your retina) to make tiny little "burns." This has been very carefully studied and can stop or slow down the rate of eye damage in the future. It is not entirely known how it works, but one theory is that it improves the blood supply to the rest of your retina, and so your body stops making the new lining cells and new blood vessels that cause the problems. Every tiny laser burn forms a little scar. They fire these laser burns mostly around the outside of your retina so that you may not see so well out of the corners of your eyes, but they are trying to protect the important central part of your vision. You will likely get several sessions of laser therapy so that over time you will be given a few thousand little burns. This produces several thousand little scars. Scar tissue does not need much blood, oxygen, or nutrients, and so the rest of your retina gets more of those things and is able to stay healthier.

What is a vitrectomy?

If eye damage progresses, it can cause several problems. If the fragile new blood vessels burst, they can bleed into the vitreous (the clear liquid at the center of the eye). The blood clot in the vitreous is opaque, and so light cannot pass through it to get to your retina. If the new blood vessels become scarred and start to contract, they can pull the retina off the back of your eye and cause it to be distorted.

The retina is shaped like a TV or satellite reception disc. Imagine if someone took a hammer to your TV satellite dish and bent the smooth surface into a lumpy mess. Your TV reception would not be good at all. The same thing can happen if fibrous scars mess up your retina. A vitrectomy is a surgical operation where a skilled eye surgeon goes in and sucks all of the blood clot from your vitreous and replaces it with clear fluid again. The surgeon may also cut and remove the fibrous scars and use laser beams to help keep your retina pinned back in the normal position again.

If I have diabetic retinopathy, should I stop taking aspirin?

If you have had a recent bleed into your eye, then you should not be taking aspirin. However, several large, well-controlled research studies have shown that there is no need to stop taking aspirin just because you have been told you have diabetic retinopathy. Unless you have had a recent bleed, the benefits of taking aspirin most likely outweigh the risks. You should talk to your doctor about this.

Apart from getting regular eye exams, what else can I do to prevent eye damage?

There are several things you can do to lower your risk of getting diabetic eye damage. The most important is to work to get your blood glucose control as close to normal as you can. An important research study called the Diabetes Control and Complications Trial (DCCT) looked at this in over 1,400 young people with type 1 diabetes. Half of them kept their HbA1c at around 7.0 percent for over six years, while the other half kept the HbA1c at around 9.0 percent during this time. There was much less eye damage in the group who kept the HbA1c closer to normal. In fact, some of those patients who already had diabetic eye damage at the start of the DCCT had less diabetic eye damage six or more years later, which seems truly remarkable. If you have diabetes and you smoke, then quitting smoking will decrease your risk of getting eye damage. Taking ACE-inhibitor drugs will also decrease your risk for eye damage.

Chapter 10

Preventing Kidney Damage

- How does a high blood glucose damage the kidneys?
- Does everybody with diabetes get kidney damage eventually?
- If I have diabetes, will I end up needing dialysis?
- What is the difference between hemodialysis and peritoneal dialysis?
- Can someone with diabetes get a kidney transplant?
- What can I do to lower my risk of getting kidney damage?
- What kind of diet can help prevent kidney damage?
- What is microalbuminuria?
- Why does having kidney damage increase my risk of heart disease?

How does a high blood glucose damage the kidneys?

We don't know all of the ways that high blood glucose levels can damage the kidneys. The kidneys are one of the main filtering systems in your body. They work to filter chemicals out of your blood so that you retain the correct amounts of water, electrolytes, protein, and other important substances. High levels of glucose seem to "gum up" this filtering system. In the first few years of someone having diabetes, the kidneys can actually increase in size slightly and seem to be able to filter even better than a non-diabetic person's kidney. The kidney contains lots of little filtering units (called nephrons). Over time the filtering membrane of these nephrons gets thickened and leaky. They begin to allow small amounts of protein to leak out into the urine. A strange protein called amyloid gets deposited in the nephrons. They become scarred. Eventually, the kidneys stop being able to get rid of important chemicals from the body. A substance called creatinine starts to build up in your blood. The blood pressure starts to rise. Eventually, the kidneys start to fail so that the person needs kidney dialysis or a kidney transplant in order to stay healthy.

Does everybody with diabetes get kidney damage eventually?

No, some people never get kidney damage, even after having diabetes for several decades. In fact, if you have had diabetes for twenty years and show no signs of kidney damage, then it is unlikely that you ever will. Most people with diabetes who are going to have kidney problems will show signs in the first ten years. Although part of this is related to how high your blood glucose average is over years, there must be other things going on. In some families where several members have diabetes, none of them get kidney damage, while other families have several members with diabetes, and all of them get kidney damage. This suggests that genetic factors offer protection to the filtering units of the kidneys in some families.

If I have diabetes, will I end up needing kidney dialysis?

Not necessarily. If you do show signs of kidney damage from your diabetes, there are a lot of things that can be done to slow down or stop the damage so that you may never need dialysis.

What is the difference between hemodialysis and peritoneal dialysis?

Kidney dialysis is a way to help clean toxins out of your blood when your own kidneys are not able to do that effectively on their own. If you get hemodialysis, then a surgeon inserts an artificial connecting tube between an artery and vein in your arm to make it easier to hook you up to the dialysis machine. You go into a dialysis center two or three times a week. They connect you to a machine that takes blood out of your artery and passes it through a membrane filter that removes toxins from your blood. The "cleaned up" blood is then passed back into your vein. You will stay hooked up for four or five hours and then go home.

With peritoneal dialysis you have a small device placed in the wall of your abdomen to allow you to run fluid into the space in your abdomen between all of your guts and other organs. You get trained how to hook yourself up to a large bag of fluid every night. There are a variety of different techniques that are used. You run the fluid into your abdomen for several hours. Toxins can pass out of your body into the fluid. A few hours later, you can drain the fluid out again. How often you need to run in fluid and drain it again varies.

If your kidneys are not working properly and your doctor thinks that dialysis would be a good option for you, then a kidney specialist (a nephrologist) can explain all the options in detail. The advantage of hemodialysis is that it gets rid of more toxins over a shorter period of time, so you only need to come in two or three times a week. With peritoneal dialysis, you can do more of it at home, but you usually need to do it at least once a day. Although dialysis can be quite a hassle, most people feel a lot better when they get the toxins cleaned out of their blood. Even if you would prefer to get a kidney transplant, you may need to do dialysis for several months or more while waiting for a kidney to become available.

Can someone with diabetes get a kidney transplant?

Yes. In fact, diabetes is the most common reason for kidney transplants nowadays. While there are lots of things that can be done to protect you from getting severe kidney damage, if you do develop kidney failure and need a transplant, the results of kidney transplantation are usually excellent for people with diabetes. The surgeon will usually leave your own two kidneys where they are. Even if they don't work as well as they should, they are still doing some filtering. Your new kidney will be put in your pelvis and attached to your bladder.

What can I do to lower my risk of getting kidney damage?

There are four things that will dramatically reduce your chance of getting diabetic kidney damage (which is called diabetic nephropathy). The most important, if you have diabetes and you smoke, is to quit smoking. For reasons that are not entirely clear, the blood vessels supplying blood to your kidneys get damaged easily by the effects of smoking. Kidneys deteriorate at least four times faster among people with diabetes who smoke compared with people with diabetes who don't smoke. Improving your blood glucose control also helps slow down the rate of diabetic kidney damage. If you can work to get your HbA1c under 7.0 percent and can keep it there, this helps tremendously. Improving your blood pressure to below 130/80 is another thing that helps. And even if your blood pressure is normal, taking an ACE-inhibitor drug or an ACE receptor blocking drug gives your kidneys tremendous protection.

What kind of diet can help prevent kidney damage?

For most people with diabetes, the best diet is one that gives you most of your calories from unrefined, high-fiber carbohydrate, with modest amounts of healthy protein and fat. If you have high blood pressure, you may be asked to reduce your salt intake. If you are developing kidney damage, you may be asked to reduce the amount of protein in your diet even more than usual. One of the worries that many doctors have about people with diabetes eating low carb/high protein diets (like the Atkins diet) is that this diet is not good for your kidneys.

What is microalbuminuria?

If you are spilling tiny amounts of protein from your kidneys, this is called microalbuminuria. Like most great big, complicated medical words, it is straightforward to understand if you break it down. *Micro* means small. The most important protein that we measure is called albumen. So if we find small amounts of *albumen* in your urine, we combine those three words and call it *micro-albumin-uria*.

If you are spilling small amounts of protein, you would not know it. Your urine will not look or smell any different. Nowadays there are cheap, simple, and sensitive laboratory tests to detect microalbuminuria. If you have diabetes, you should be getting this test done every year. Microalbuminuria can be detected many years before you would ever know that there is a problem in your kidneys. This gives your health care team plenty of time to help you to do things to slow down or stop the damage.

Why does having kidney damage increase my risk of heart disease?

It is not known why this is true, but it is. It may be that if your kidneys are damaged from diabetes, this is a sign that the linings of your blood vessels are just vulnerable to damage from blood glucose not only in your kidneys, but elsewhere, too. I sometimes think of microalbuminuria as being like the "canary in the coal mine" for heart disease. You probably know that story. In olden days, coal miners used to bring canaries down the mine with them in cages. These tiny birds were much more sensitive to the presence of poisonous gases like carbon monoxide. If the canary keeled over and died, the miners knew that there was poisonous gas in the mine, and so they could get out quick and then do something to clear the air in the mine. If people with diabetes start spilling even small amounts of protein in their urine, it tells me that I need to help them do things to reduce their risk of heart disease, as well as do things to protect their kidneys.

Chapter 11

Nerve Damage: Feet and Legs

- How does a high blood glucose cause damage to the nerves (neuropathy)?
- Are there different kinds of neuropathy?
- How would I know if I had neuropathy?
- What causes the burning pain in my feet?
- Why is the pain in my feet worse at nighttime?
- How do I know that my painful symptoms are due to diabetes?
- What can I do to lower my risk of getting diabetic neuropathy?
- Why does neuropathy pain get worse when you improve your blood glucose?
- What can I do for burning pain in my feet?
- Are there creams to treat neuropathy?
- What are the best drugs to treat neuropathy?
- Do these drugs heal the nerves or just dull the pain?
- What other treatments can help the pain from neuropathy?
- If I lose the sensation in my feet, does that mean I will end up needing an amputation?
- If I have lost the sensation in my feet, will I ever get it back?
- If I have lost the sensation in my feet, how can I protect them?
- Why should I take my shoes and socks off every time I go to see my doctor?
- What is gangrene?
- What is a Charcot foot?

How does a high blood glucose cause damage to the nerves (neuropathy)?

Nerves are among the most unusual cells in your body. The nerve at the tip of your toe is made up of a whole bunch of tiny, thin, and very long cells that stretch all the way from the tip of your toe to the spinal cord in your back. So that single cell could be several feet long! That makes it vulnerable to damage from high blood glucose levels. If the glucose cannot be metabolized properly inside the nerves, a substance called sorbitol can build up inside and cause the nerve to stop working properly.

Nerves are a bit like electrical wires. Some are thicker than others; some are insulated, while others are bare. When the glucose level is too high for a number of years, the covering of those nerves (a substance called myelin that acts like an insulating sheath around some of your nerves) can get damaged and may disappear. This makes it harder for the nerve cells to send signals so fast. They get "inflamed" and may start firing off signals on their own.

Are there different kinds of diabetic neuropathy?

Yes. You have many different types of nerve in your body, and all of them can get damaged from diabetes. Think of the nerves in your body as the electrical wires running throughout your house. The problems you get will depend on which wires get damaged. In your house, if a leak into your attic caused a short circuit in the wires up there, the heater or light in your bathroom might stop working. If a mouse in the basement chewed through the electrical wire to your washing machine, then that appliance would stop working. In a similar way, the problems you get from nerve damage depend on which particular nerves get damaged.

The term diabetic neuropathy simply means "damage to the nerves due to diabetes." The nerves in your feet are often the ones that get damaged first, probably because those are the longest nerves in your body. Some nerves supply your sweat glands. If they get damaged, you will get dry feet. This can lead to cracked skin and may allow bacteria to get under your skin, causing infection. Other nerves send signals of pain or heat to your brain. So if you stand on a piece of broken glass or touch a hot radiator, those nerves tell your brain about it, and you quickly do something about it. So if those pain and heat sensitive nerves get damaged, it can cause a big problem for you because you may not notice that you are being injured.

Nerves also supply your muscles and tell them when to contract. If those nerves get damaged, your muscles will become weaker, and your bones and joints may move into unhealthy positions. Nerves also help your stomach and guts and heart and blood pressure to work properly without you ever thinking about it. If those nerves get damaged, it can lead to problems. Many thousands of nerve fibers get bundled together inside your body. If the tiny little blood vessel that supplies that bundle of nerves gets blocked because of diabetes, this can cause another type of neuropathy.

How would I know if I had neuropathy?

Because your nerves do so many things all throughout your body, you may get a wide variety of symptoms. If the nerves supplying your pain and heat sensors get damaged, they may start "misfiring" on their own so that you feel as if your feet are burning or on fire. Your skin may become super-sensitive, so that even the soft touch of the sheets on your bed seems to sting and tingle. You may feel stabbing or burning pain like needles being poked into your feet. If the nerves supplying your sweat glands get damaged, you may notice that your feet are dry and cracked. You may notice that some of your muscles are weaker than they used to be. The muscles around your eyelid and eyeball have tiny nerves helping them to work. Damage to one of them can sometimes cause double vision. If the nerves supplying your stomach get damaged, you may notice that you feel bloated, even after eating quite small meals. If the nerves that help keep your blood pressure up get damaged, you may feel dizzy when you stand up too quickly. For a man with diabetes, damage to the nerves supplying your penis can cause erectile dysfunction.

One of the biggest problems with nerve damage from diabetes is that it can come on so slowly and quietly that you may not get any symptoms at all. If the nerves supplying your feet get damaged, you may just gradually lose sensation in them. Your feet become numb so that you feel no pain in them at all. Although you might think that this is a good thing, it really isn't.

If things are working normally and you stand on a nail, the pain sensors in your skin send a signal to your brain in a fraction of a second saying, "Help, there is an unpleasant stabbing pain down here!" You immediately pull your foot away from the nail, inspect your foot, and then do something to help it to heal up. But if that signal does not arrive in your brain because the wiring is so rusty and broken that it doesn't conduct the electrical message anymore, then you do nothing about the nail sticking into your foot. Hours or days later, it might get infected, and your foot might start to swell up or to smell bad; and so then you detect that there is a problem. But by then, it has become a huge problem. If you had detected it right away, you could have prevented a huge problem.

You should expect that your doctor or someone else on your health care team will inspect your feet at least once a year, and test the skin on the bottom of your feet to see if you can feel things normally. They won't stick nails into your feet, I hope, but they will test to see if you can feel vibration or the light touch of a piece of plastic.

What causes the burning pain in my feet?

The sensation of burning heat and prickly, stabbing pain in your feet can be really unpleasant and exhausting. This can come on quite suddenly and last for weeks or months unless it is treated. It often starts after your blood glucose levels have been very high for several days or more. Sometimes burning pain in the feet is the first symptom that makes people go to see their doctor, where they find out that they have diabetes. Or maybe you had fairly mild diabetes and had no pain in your feet, but then you get a bad chest infection and have really high blood glucose levels for a few weeks. The next thing you know, your feet are burning, and you can hardly sleep.

This kind of diabetic neuropathy is usually caused because the covering of your nerves (the myelin sheath that acts a bit like the plastic insulation on a wire) gets damaged from the high blood glucose levels and shrivels up. When the covering goes off your nerves, they stop conducting properly. They become inflamed, and they start "firing off" on their own and sending signals to your brain to say, "Help, it is burning hot down here!"—even though there is nothing actually causing heat to the skin of your feet.

Although this is very unpleasant for you while you have these symptoms, one good thing about this type of diabetic neuropathy is that the nerves themselves are still alive and working. It is the covering to them that has peeled off. If you can get your blood glucose levels back down to near normal and keep them there, then the nerves can heal up. In fact, they can regrow the insulating myelin sheath around them and become as good as new again.

Why is the pain in my feet worse at nighttime?

It really seems unfair. You have been suffering the discomfort in your feet all day long and are finally home, done with the work and hassles of the day and looking forward to a nice rest. But as you lie quietly in bed, you find that the burning pain and discomfort in your feet is getting worse rather than better. Even the touch of your bedclothes drives you nuts and sets off a wave of stabbing, prickly, burning pain. This happens because, during the day, you have a million things that you have to concentrate on as you dress yourself, eat your food, walk to work, talk to your friends and co-workers, answer the telephone, and so forth. The part of your brain that is designed to focus on how your feet are feeling gets distracted because other parts of your brain are working overtime to help you get through all of your daily chores.

But at nighttime, when you are lying in a quiet, dark room with no distractions, your brain starts to focus on how your feet are feeling. As a result, it seems that the pain gets much worse. Some people find that if they get up and walk around the room, rub their feet, make a cup of tea, or read a book, this helps to take their mind off the pain in their feet, but as soon as they stop those activities and lie quietly again, the pain gets worse.

How do I know that my painful symptoms are due to diabetes?

If you have pains in your feet or in other parts of your body, you should go see your doctor to figure out what is causing your symptoms. Other things can cause damage to the nerves. If you are not getting enough vitamins in your diet, especially the B-group vitamins (thiamine, riboflavin, folic acid, and vitamin B12), you can get severe damage to your nerves. If you have an underactive thyroid gland and don't produce enough thyroid hormone, your nerves will stop working properly. There are some diseases that cause inflammation in your blood vessels and joints that can damage the nerves, too. Drinking too much alcohol is unhealthy for your nerves. Your doctor can usually figure out the cause of your neuropathy by talking to you, examining you, and taking some blood tests.

What can I do to lower my risk of getting diabetic neuropathy?

Eat a healthy diet that contains a variety of food and vitamins. Taking a multivitamin that contains 100 percent of the recommended daily amount of the B vitamins is sensible. Do not drink alcohol to excess. This means no more than one alcoholic drink per day for women and no more than two alcoholic drinks per day for men. In fact, it would be a good idea to stop drinking alcohol altogether for a month to see if your painful symptoms improve.

The most important thing you can do is whatever it takes to bring your blood glucose level as close to normal as possible and keep it there for several months. Several research studies have shown that if you can keep your HbA1c below 7.0 percent, then your risk of getting neuropathy is very much lower. And if you already have painful diabetic neuropathy, getting your HbA1c below 7.0 percent can help the nerves to heal.

Why does neuropathy pain get worse when you improve your blood glucose?

This can be very frustrating. You are doing everything you can to help yourself. You are eating healthy, drinking no alcohol, taking vitamins, and keeping your blood glucose close to normal. But instead of the pains in your feet getting better, they seem to be worse. This can happen, especially in the first few weeks of improved blood glucose control. This is probably because your damaged nerves are beginning to recover and regrow the myelin sheath around them. They start to "wake up" and send signals up and down their length. Your brain is suddenly getting more vigorous signals from those nerves. The good news is that if you keep your blood glucose down, then your nerves will continue to heal, and the painful symptoms will go away.

What can I do for burning pain in my feet?

You will hear all sorts of folk remedies for aching, painful feet. Well-intentioned friends and neighbors may suggest wrapping them in dock leaves or bathing them in Epsom salts. Most of those folk remedies are harmless, and some of them may help. Massaging the feet can give some relief, and soaking them in cool or tepid (but not hot) water might help.

Are there creams to treat neuropathy?

Yes. The best creams are those that contain capsaicin. Capsaicin is the active ingredient in hot peppers like jalapenos. If you eat too much of a hot pepper, it can burn your tongue and then make it go numb. Applying capsaicin cream to your painful feet can work the same way. It is best to wear plastic gloves when applying capsaicin to prevent it from making your hands go numb. If the pain is bothering you at nighttime, then carefully wash and dry your feet before you go to bed, and then rub the cream onto your skin over the painful area. Put clean socks on your feet to help keep the cream in contact with the skin and to prevent it from being rubbed off by the bedclothes.

Capsaicin cream comes in different strengths (0.025%, 0.075%). I suggest starting at a low strength and using a higher strength if the low dose doesn't help. Capsaicin cream might sting or cause a prickly sensation at first. That usually goes away in a few minutes. If the pain wakes you later in the night, you should remove the cotton socks, apply more cream, and put the socks back on again. You can apply capsaicin cream two or three times a day. It is most effective if the burning and painful area is quite small. Sometimes capsaicin cream will give you enough relief by itself. If not, it can be combined with pills.

What are the best drugs to treat neuropathy?

One of the most effective drugs to treat painful neuropathy is an old-fashioned kind of drug that can also treat depression. These are the tricyclic antidepressants such as amitriptyline, nortriptyline, and desipramine. The dose of these drugs needed to treat depression is often 100–150 mg per day, but much lower doses can be very effective to help the pain of neuropathy. I usually start at just 10 mg or 25 mg taken at bedtime. The drugs work by "turning down the volume" in the area of your brain that is receiving the pain signals from your nerves. They can make you feel a bit drowsy and cause dry mouth and blurred vision in some people, especially at higher doses. They may not be suitable for people with certain heart or bladder conditions.

Funnily enough, the more modern and popular antidepressant drugs (the selective serotonin reuptake inhibitors, or SSRIs), like fluoxetine (Prozac) and sertraline (Zoloft), are not effective in treating painful neuropathy. However, a combined serotonin and norepinephrine reuptake inhibitor, duloxetine (Cymbalta), has been shown to be effective in randomized clinical trials. Many other types of drugs can be tried. The fact that so many different ones are used tells you that their effects are unpredictable. Sometimes they work really well on one person but don't help someone else. Drugs to treat seizure disorders are sometimes helpful. These include carbamazepine and phenytoin.

The most widely prescribed drugs for painful neuropathy are gabapentin (Neurontin) or pregabalin (Lyrica). In my experience, these are less effective than the tricyclic antidepressants, but they work well on some people. They are more expensive and have different side effects, including dizziness and confusion. Sometimes combinations of more than one type of drug may be needed to help give you relief of your symptoms. It is important to see a doctor who is experienced in treating nerve pain.

Do these drugs heal the nerves or just dull the pain?

The drugs mentioned above are really just working to dull the pain. They make it more bearable while you wait for your nerves to heal up and for the pain to go away. The good news is that painful neuropathy almost always goes away on its own eventually, although it can take twelve to eighteen months in some cases.

Attempts to heal neuropathy have not been successful so far. A substance called sorbitol builds up inside damaged nerves. Drugs called aldose reductase inhibitors have been used to lower sorbitol levels, but they have a lot of side effects and have not improved how the nerves work. The ACE-inhibitor drugs that help protect against heart disease, kidney damage, and eye damage from diabetes may also help protect your nerves against neuropathy. Alpha-lipoic acid has also been shown to help heal nerves a small amount.

What other treatments can help the pain from neuropathy?

If you put an electrical stimulation on the skin for thirty minutes a day for several weeks using a device called a Transcutaneous Electrical Nerve Stimulation (TENS) unit, this can improve the pain of neuropathy. It can be used on its own or along with pills to dull the pain. Magnets have also been used, either as insoles in your shoes or as inserts in the sheets covering your mattress. Like so many alternative therapies, there have been very few well-controlled research trials testing whether magnets are really effective or not.

One of my patients actually got a foot ulcer as a result of wearing magnetic insoles in her shoes. The insoles were smooth on one side but had lots of little raised bumps on the other side. She wore the magnetic insoles with the bumpy part next to her skin. The pressure from this punched a hole through her skin and caused an ulcer that became infected and caused a serious problem.

If I lose the sensation in my feet, does that mean I will end up needing an amputation?

Very, very few people with diabetes need to get their toes or feet or legs amputated nowadays. Although having neuropathy puts your feet at risk of injury, there is a lot that you can do to protect them. Also, if a problem is detected early, there are excellent treatments that can heal those injuries. Almost all of the diabetic patients that I see who need to get part of their leg amputated are people who smoke cigarettes and have really poor circulation to their feet and people who waited too long before seeing their doctor.

If I have lost the sensation in my feet, will I ever get it back?

Although this does happen occasionally, it is not common. When the nerves begin to get damaged from high blood glucose, it often causes pain. The myelin nerve sheaths shrivel up, but the nerve cell is still alive and able to heal with improved blood glucose control and healthy diet and vitamins. But once the nerve damage continues and the nerve dies, the pain often goes away so that the feet, legs, and sometimes even the hands become numb and lose all sensation. It is not likely that those nerves will ever work again, so the sensation in your feet is not likely to come back.

If I have lost the sensation in my feet, how can I protect them?

If you smoke, then quitting smoking is the most important thing you can do to protect your feet. Smoking reduces the circulation to your feet tremendously. It increases your risk of getting severe damage that might require amputation of part of your leg. You should continue to eat a healthy diet and work to keep your blood glucose as close to normal as possible.

Use common sense to protect your feet from damage. Remember, you will not be able to feel it if you step on a tack or a piece of glass, so avoid walking around barefoot, and make sure you test the temperature of bathwater before putting your feet into it. It is best to avoid using heating pads or hot water bottles. Almost all causes of foot ulcers, infections, and amputations begin as a minor injury that could have been avoided. When trimming your nails, do not cut them too close to the toe. Trim them to the shape of the toe (not straight across), and buff them with a nail file. You want to avoid leaving sharp corners or edges. Another common cause of an ulcer is when a sharp corner of nail from one toe gets pressed into the toe next to it in tight-fitting shoes.

Use lukewarm water and mild soap to wash your feet. If the feet are dry, use a moisturizing lotion on them. Check your feet every day for any signs of injury or skin breaks of blisters or hot areas or athlete's foot fungus infection. If you can't see the underside of your feet, you should use a mirror or have someone else look for you. Use socks that are loose-fitting and will wick away moisture (so cotton rather than nylon is best).

Choose shoes that are well-fitting but not too tight. They should allow enough room around your toes. If your feet are oddly shaped, you may need to see a podiatrist (a foot-care specialist) to get shoes and insoles that are custom made to protect your feet. You should expect your doctor or nurse to examine your feet at every visit. You should ask to have this done and take your shoes and socks or stockings off when you are in the doctor's office to make it easier.

If you follow all of these pieces of advice you are very likely to avoid serious problems with your feet.

Why should I take my shoes and socks off every time I go to see my doctor?

If you do have neuropathy and have lost the ability to feel it when you walk on a pebble or piece of glass or a nail, then you are at great danger of injuring your feet. If you have neuropathy, it is important to examine your own feet every day and to ask for your doctor to do a more detailed check of your feet when you come for an appointment. But some medical offices have taken this to extremes. There are notices everywhere telling you that if you have diabetes, you must take your shoes and socks off at every visit. Sometimes the medical assistant or nurse who puts you in the room will insist that you are barefoot before the doctor comes in to see you.

Many of my patients object to this and find it to be demeaning to their intelligence. I can totally understand their attitude. If you are young and healthy and have good diabetes control and know for sure that you have perfectly normal sensation in your feet, then it does not make sense to take your shoes and socks off every single time you come in. Maybe you were in just a week or two before and had a full foot exam then and were told that everything was healthy, but now the nurse is insisting that you take your shoes and socks off again. You can always refuse, of course, but sometimes it is not worth fighting the system. If the nurse or medical assistant is on a mission to make sure that all patients with diabetes have to get their shoes and socks removed at every visit, they may get very annoyed with you for trying to bend "the rules."

What is gangrene?

This is one of the most dreaded terms that you will hear. It brings on visions of soldiers with battlefield injuries who can't get help soon enough, and so "gangrene sets in." It is an old-fashioned term that means "dead tissue." It occurs when the blood supply to your toes or your foot gets cut off so that the muscle and bones and tendons are starved of oxygen and nutrients. Usually the toe or foot will shrivel up and turn black. If it gets infected with certain bacteria, it can become wet and black and may even have gas bubbles develop under the skin.

Gangrene is very serious and usually means that the toe or foot will need to be amputated before it spreads infection into your bloodstream. If you develop a deep, uncomfortable pain in a toe or foot and it turns cold and blue, you need to see a doctor as soon as possible (within hours). Sometimes surgery can be done to improve the circulation and save the foot, but if it is left too long and turns black, then amputation is the only treatment option.

What is a Charcot foot?

You usually think of neuropathy causing damage to the nerves that supply you with pain and heat sensation, but nerves also supply your muscles. Your foot is made up of several small bones that line up with each other to give your foot the nice, curved shape that you are used to. If the nerves to the small muscles of the feet get damaged, the bones may collapse or crack and break. If you have damage to the nerves that supply pain sensation, you might not even notice the pain from the collapsed or broken bones, but the foot will look different than it used to and will feel warm to the touch because of all the inflammation from the damage. Doctors call this a Charcot foot (named after the famous French neurologist Jean-Martin Charcot, who described the condition). You should go to see your doctor if you notice that your arch has collapsed or your foot has changed shape or is hot to the touch.

Chapter 12

NERVE DAMAGE: LESS COMMON FORMS

- Why do my fingers feel swollen when I try to make a fist?
- What is carpal tunnel syndrome?
- Why is carpal tunnel syndrome more common in people with diabetes?
- How can carpal tunnel syndrome be treated?
- Is erectile dysfunction inevitable for men with diabetes?
- How do I explain erectile dysfunction to my spouse or partner?
- What can be done to treat erectile dysfunction?
- What is gastroparesis?
- How would I know if I had gastroparesis?
- What treatments are available for gastroparesis?
- Why do some people with diabetes have bad breath?
- Can diabetes cause diarrhea or constipation?

Why do my fingers feel swollen when I try to make a fist?

Several things could cause this. The only way to know for sure is to go see your doctor and let her or him examine you. The most common reason that your fingers swell up is because there is too much water being held in the soft tissue around your bones, tendons, joints, and muscles. The medical term for water being held in soft tissue so that it swells up is edema. A number of drugs can cause this as a side effect. The diabetes drugs rosiglitazone (Avandia) and pioglitazone (Actos) can do this.

Sometimes insulin can cause edema. This is especially likely if you have had high blood glucose levels for several weeks and then increase your insulin dose a lot to try to bring the blood glucose down. Swollen fingers could also happen if you were allergic to a drug. It could also happen if your joints become inflamed because of arthritis. Another common cause of stiff, swollen hands is carpal tunnel syndrome.

What is carpal tunnel syndrome?

Your wrist is made up of a number of small bones held close together. The medical term for this is carpus. On the front of your wrist (the same side as the palm of your hand), a lot of important things pass from your arm into your hand. These include tendons connecting the muscles in your forearm with your fingers, blood vessels to supply your hand with nutrients, and a nerve called the median nerve. This nerve helps part of your hand to feel pain and also helps the muscles near your thumb to work properly. All of these blood vessels, tendons, and nerves pass in front of the wrist bones (the carpal bones). A tight band of fibrous tissue passes in front of the nerves, blood vessels, and tendons, enclosing them in a tight tunnel (called the carpal tunnel). If the tunnel gets too tight (perhaps because your wrist swells with fluid), then the median nerve can get trapped, crushed, and damaged. This can cause pain in your hand and forearm and weakness in the thumb muscles. The symptoms are often worse when you wake up in the morning and get better during the day, but they can also get worse if you have to use your hands and fingers a lot at your work.

Why is carpal tunnel syndrome more common in people with diabetes?

If your nerves are damaged from high blood glucose levels, they may be more inflamed and fragile than normal. If the median nerve is already damaged from diabetes, even a small amount of extra pressure in the carpal tunnel can push it "over the edge." Poor diabetes control and some of the drugs used to treat diabetes can sometimes cause you to retain fluid. When fluid builds up in the tissues under the skin, we call that edema. Diabetes makes it more likely that your carpal tunnel will get tighter and makes your median nerve more vulnerable to the pressure from that tightness, and so carpal tunnel syndrome is more common in people with diabetes.

How can carpal tunnel syndrome be treated?

Sometimes your doctor will order nerve conduction tests to be sure that you do have carpal tunnel syndrome. This is a test where they put electrodes on your forearm and hand to test how fast the nerves conduct the electric stimulus. That test can feel a bit unpleasant, because they give you small electrical shocks. To treat carpal tunnel syndrome, your doctor may give you an injection into your wrist to reduce the swelling in the carpal tunnel. If that relieves your painful symptoms, then they might try giving you a wrist brace to wear to take the pressure off your wrist to see if that will relieve the pressure and allow your nerve to heal. If those things don't work, you may be sent to a surgeon who can cut the band of fibrous tissue in front of your wrist to relieve the pressure in your carpal tunnel permanently.

Is erectile dysfunction inevitable for men with diabetes?

Not at all, especially if you can keep your blood glucose levels close to normal, eat a healthy diet, and avoid drinking alcohol to excess. But over half of all men over fifty with diabetes experience some degree of erectile dysfunction. Even though they have interest in sex and are in a healthy, happy relationship, their erection becomes gradually softer and does not stay hard for as long as it used to. There are a lot of reasons for this. A normal erection requires lots of things to work well. You need to feel relaxed and unstressed. The nerves supplying the penis need to be healthy, and the blood supply to the penis needs to work well. If you are stressed and worried that you might not be able to get an erection, that can upset the process. This is sometimes called *performance anxiety*, because worrying that you won't be able to get an erection that is stiff enough to allow you to perform sexual intercourse can turn a slight problem into a major one very quickly.

If the nerves are damaged from diabetes, they may not give the correct signals to the blood vessels to let more blood into your penis and prevent blood from leaking out again. And if you have narrowing of the arteries supplying your penis, then not enough blood can get through to cause an erection. Any combination of these problems can cause erectile dysfunction. Hormone problems such as low testosterone levels or high prolactin levels can also occur, but these are not a common cause of erectile dysfunction in men with diabetes. Your doctor should be able to figure out what the main problem is for you by talking to you, examining you, and doing a few simple laboratory tests.

How do I explain erectile dysfunction to my spouse or partner?

This can be awkward and embarrassing and difficult, even if you have a good relationship and are good at communicating with your spouse or partner. You can certainly ask your partner to come with you to a doctor's appointment and ask your doctor to explain it to both of you.

Here are some of the things that you should explain to your partner. Your erectile dysfunction is not your partner's fault. You still find your partner attractive. It is not your fault either. You are no less of a man because you have erectile dysfunction. Usually erectile dysfunction is not caused by a low testosterone level in men with diabetes (but your doctor will check to make sure). It is usually caused because the delicate nerves that cause blood to flow into your penis to make it stiffer have become damaged from diabetes.

There are several treatments that can help. If you feel tense and under pressure to perform, your erectile dysfunction will get worse, so if you and your partner stay relaxed and good humored about it, things will go better. If you find other ways to give each other sensual pleasure without being under pressure to have sexual intercourse every time, this will help. Counselors at sexual dysfunction clinics often have specific techniques for you to try that can really help.

What can be done to treat erectile dysfunction?

A group of drugs called phosphodiesterase-5 inhibitors has revolutionized the treatment of erectile dysfunction. The three main drugs in the group, sildenafil (Viagra), vardenafil (Levitra), and tadalafil (Cialis), have become household names. They are heavily advertised during televised sporting events like football and baseball! These drugs all act in the same way but vary in how quickly they begin to work and how long the effect lasts. They help the blood vessel supplying blood to the penis to open up, allowing blood in faster than it drains out, and so the penis becomes stiffer for longer. Because they cause the blood vessels to dilate, they can cause headaches, flushing, and runny nose as side effects. If you have heart disease and are taking nitrates, they may not be safe. They can sometimes cause problems with your vision, and if they work too well, can cause the penis to stay so stiff and engorged for hours on end that it can cause pain and damage to the penis (this condition is called priapism).

All of these drugs work well for most men with diabetes who have erectile dysfunction. If they do not work, or if you are not able to take them because of side effects, then there are other options. An injection of papaverine or phentolamine or alprostadil given into the base of the penis can cause an erection sufficient to allow intercourse. This is obviously a bit more painful and awkward than simply taking a pill but can be quite effective. Sometimes two of the drugs can be used together. Alprostadil can also be given by pushing a thin tube up the penis and injecting the drug from inside.

More mechanical solutions include vacuum devices to pull more blood into the penis until it is enlarged and stiff enough to allow intercourse. This is followed by placing a rubber band around the base of the penis to keep the penis stiff during intercourse. If the erectile dysfunction is due to a poor blood supply to the penis, then surgery to improve the blood supply can be successful. Plastic implants can also be inserted inside the penis to keep it stiff enough for intercourse.

Since the introduction of the phosphodiesterase-5 inhibitors a few years ago, it is much less common to need to use the alternative treatment that I have described. Your doctor can go over these options in more detail or can refer you to a sexual dysfunction specialist.

What is gastroparesis?

This medical term means "sluggish stomach" or maybe "flabby, weak-muscled stomach." To understand why that can happen, let me explain a bit about how your stomach works. The stomach is like a stretchy bag with openings at both ends. There are muscles woven into the walls of the bag and other muscles wrapped tightly around each end of the bag to keep it closed. For those muscles to work properly, tiny little nerves, called autonomic nerves, need to be working properly.

When food first arrives, the tight muscles at either end keep the bag closed. The muscles in the wall of the stomach contract and relax over and over to slosh the food around. This gets it mixed up with acid and stomach juices that begin to break the food up. Once the food is well mixed up and partly broken down, then the tight muscles at the bottom end of the stomach should open, and the muscles lining the walls begin to squeeze the food gradually out into the rest of your guts, where it gets absorbed.

If those tiny little autonomic nerves get damaged because of high blood glucose, then the muscles in the stomach stop working properly. The muscles lining the walls get weak and stretched so that the bag gets bigger, and the food just sits there for much longer.

How would I know if I had gastroparesis?

When your stomach muscles get flabby and weak, it can cause some unpleasant symptoms. You may feel bloated, even after small meals. You might even be able to feel and hear that there is food sloshing around down there. It can cause you to belch up unpleasant smelling gas and be embarrassing socially. One of the problems with gastroparesis is that how severe it is can vary a lot from day to day. Some days your stomach empties faster than others, and so your blood glucose readings can become very unpredictable.

If you took a large dose of insulin before your meal because you ate a lot of carbohydrate in it, you might get a really low blood glucose an hour after the meal, because the insulin has "kicked in," but the food is still stuck in your stomach. Your blood glucose will only rise once the carbohydrate has left the stomach and been broken down into glucose inside your small intestines. If it gets held up in your stomach for longer than usual, the insulin shot that you took before the meal will push your blood glucose down below normal. But then a couple of hours later, your sluggish stomach might finally release all of that food into your small intestines, and so your blood glucose will go up really high. So even if you do not feel the symptoms of bloating, fullness, belching, or bad breath, if your blood glucose readings are becoming very unpredictable for reasons that you can't explain, then gastroparesis might be the problem.

It is possible to diagnose gastroparesis by using advanced tests in which they give you a meal of solid and liquid food that has had small amounts of radioactive particles added to it. They can then scan your abdomen at different times after your radioactive meal to see how much of the solid and liquid food is still in your stomach and how far it has traveled down into your small intestines. Although these gastric emptying studies are interesting to look at, I rarely use them anymore with my patients. Here's why. If you have had diabetes for more than ten years, then gastric emptying studies will almost always say that your stomach does not empty properly, even if you have no symptoms of gastroparesis at all. The results of gastric emptying studies rarely help me to decide on the best treatment, either.

I have seen people with severe symptoms of gastroparesis who have gastric emptying studies that are only slightly abnormal, and I have seen other people who have terrible looking test results but only mild symptoms. So if I see people who have symptoms that sound like gastroparesis, I usually skip the fancy tests and just give them medicine that should help. If their symptoms improve in the next few weeks, then I can be confident that they had gastroparesis and that the treatment is helping. If they don't get better, then I may do tests to see if something else was causing their symptoms.

What treatments are available for gastroparesis?

There is a drug called metoclopramide (Reglan) that you can take as a pill about thirty minutes before your main meals. It stimulates the muscles lining your stomach walls to contract more vigorously and opens the muscle at the lower end so that food leaves your stomach and gets passed into your small intestines more easily. Metoclopramide can cause quite a number of side effects in some people. It can cause headaches, may make you feel drowsy, and give you a dry mouth and nose. It can also cause more serious symptoms, including some that affect your brain so that you can't stop yourself twitching and moving your arms, neck, and body. Another drug that can be very effective is erythromycin. This is mostly used as an antibiotic, and anyone who has ever had to take it as an antibiotic knows that it can cause diarrhea. This is because it stimulates the muscles in the walls of your stomach and small and large intestines to contract more vigorously. The doses used to treat infections almost always cause the bowels to speed up, causing diarrhea. But much smaller doses can help the stomach to speed up without causing diarrhea, so I often use erythromycin to help gastroparesis if metoclopramide did not work or caused too many side effects. If gastroparesis is severe and does not respond to these drugs, you may need to have surgery to help your stomach to empty better. Doctors sometimes implant an electrical pacemaker to stimulate your stomach to contract more.

Why do some people with diabetes have bad breath?

All sorts of things can cause your breath to smell bad, even if you don't have diabetes. Certain foods have a very strong smell that lingers on your breath for hours after you finish eating. Garlic, onions, and smoked fish are examples. If you don't brush and floss your teeth and keep them clean, then food can get stuck around your teeth, causing bad breath. Infections in the gums around your teeth (periodontal disease) can cause bad breath.

Periodontal disease is more common in people with diabetes and can be more severe. It is not known why, but it is possible that having high glucose levels in your blood means that your gums are sweeter; and so the bacteria that cause periodontal disease have more food to eat. High blood glucose can also make the cells that fight infection more sluggish, so they don't do as good a job of fighting the infection as they should. If you have diabetes, it is really important to make sure you get your teeth and gums checked regularly. If you have gastroparesis and food sits around in your stomach for too long, that can also cause bad breath.

Can diabetes cause diarrhea or constipation?

Yes, it can, but so can a lot of other things, so your doctor will probably do some tests before deciding if your diarrhea or constipation is because of diabetes. If your diet contains very little fiber, even if you don't have diabetes, you are more likely to have constipation. If you eat lots of fruits, vegetables, beans, and onions, you are more likely to have diarrhea. If your food or drink gets contaminated with certain bugs (bacteria and other parasites), that can cause an infection in your bowels, and that usually causes severe diarrhea.

Your small and large bowels have muscles in their walls that contract and relax in a steady rhythm when everything is working properly. Tiny autonomic nerves send signals to these muscles to tell them when to contract and relax. If these get damaged because of high blood glucose levels for many years, the large bowels stop working properly. Sometimes this can cause severe diarrhea for weeks on end. At other times it can cause constipation.

Part Three: Living with Diabetes

Chapter 13

Monitoring Blood Glucose

- Why is my fingerstick blood glucose result different from the laboratory result?
- Why do I get different numbers when I check myself on different fingers or several times in a row on the same finger?
- Why does it hurt so much when I prick my fingertips?
- Could I get skin infections from poking my fingers so much?
- Where else can I test my blood glucose?
- Are glucose readings from alternate sites just as good as fingertip results?
- Why does my doctor tell me to check my blood glucose so often but then barely glances at the results?
- Does the fasting blood glucose need to be taken at the same time every day?
- What is a continuous glucose monitor?

Why is my fingerstick blood glucose result different from the laboratory result?

Check to make sure that your blood glucose meter is working properly. Some meters come with a special "control solution" that you can use to test your meter. You put a drop of the solution onto one of your test strips, and you should get a result within a certain range. If it is between 95 and 105 mg/dL (5.3–5.8 mmol/L), for example, then your meter is working well, but if the result is below 95 or above 105, then your meter is not accurate.

Another way to test your meter is to bring it with you when you go to the laboratory for a blood test. If they are going to measure your blood glucose in the lab, you can ask for a drop of that blood to test on your meter, or you can prick your finger at the same time as the blood test and use that. Hopefully the result that you get will be close to the same as the laboratory result, but it is unlikely to be exactly the same. The machine in the laboratory might use a different testing method. The laboratory technicians probably spin your blood sample down to separate out the red blood cells from the liquid that they are floating in (which is called plasma). Your meter might test the glucose level in your whole blood (both red cells and plasma mixed together), which gives a slightly different result.

But even if the laboratory used the very same testing method and the same type of sample, you would still get slightly different results. The results should not differ by more than 10 percent, however. So if your meter gave a result of 200 mg/dL (11.1 mmol/L), then the result from the laboratory should be between 180–220 mg/dL (10–12.2 mmol/L). If it is outside of that range, then either your meter is inaccurate or maybe the problem is with the lab! That is less likely, since most laboratories do a lot of "quality control" checks.

Why do I get different numbers when I check myself on different fingers or several times in a row on the same finger?

This can be frustrating. Maybe you already know that blood glucose can go up and down during the day depending on what you eat, when you exercise, how stressed you are, and so forth. But if you prick your finger, test your blood glucose, and then immediately test it again barely one minute later—using the very same drop of blood—it would be reasonable to expect that you would get the same result. I'm afraid not.

Several things could affect the result. Maybe you didn't wash your hands and had traces of jam or sugar on your finger. Maybe the strips you used were out of date or had gone off. Maybe you forgot to calibrate your blood glucose meter or didn't get a big enough drop of blood on the strip. But truthfully, even if you did none of those things wrong and instead did everything perfectly, you will still get different results every time you test.

Although blood glucose meters are remarkably accurate little machines, they only give you an idea of what your blood glucose is. The number you get is within 5–10 percent of the true value. Let's say your actual blood glucose is 100 mg/dL. If you tested your blood ten times in a row, you might get these results: 92, 108, 103, 97, 95, 100, 105, 104, 96, 99. And if your actual blood glucose was 300 mg/dL, then the range of numbers would be even wider: 299, 328, 272, 291, 311, 301, 319, 281, 275, 325. This doesn't mean that you need to test several times and then take the average. It doesn't mean you need a more accurate meter.

Even the machines that they use in the laboratory to test your blood glucose will give you different numbers if you tested the same sample several times. But for practical purposes, it doesn't often matter whether your blood glucose is 96 or 104. Those are close to ideal for a fasting or pre-meal blood glucose. And whether your blood glucose is 291 or 325, it is a pretty high number. It is unlikely that you would do something dramatically different because it was 291 rather than 325.

Why does it hurt so much when I prick my fingertips?

Human beings use their fingers a lot! They are strong, flexible, and sensitive, so we can explore our surroundings, type, write, communicate, and hold things. In order to do all of those things, the skin covering the ends of our fingertips has a lot of nerve endings underneath. That means that it hurts more when you prick your finger than when you prick another piece of skin that has fewer nerve endings underneath. The finger-poking needles (called lancets) and the spring-loaded devices that you can get to push the lancets through the skin have been designed to do this as painlessly as possible, but it still sometimes hurts, especially if the needle strikes very close to a nerve ending (and there is no way to know that by looking at your skin). If you feel that it is really hurting more than it should, you should ask your doctor or nurse to watch you doing a finger test. Maybe you are doing it wrong. Maybe a different type of lancet or spring-loaded device would work better.

Could I get skin infections from poking my fingers so much?

It is possible but incredibly unlikely to get a skin infection from poking your fingertips with a lancet to check your blood glucose. In thirty years of being a doctor and seeing tens of thousands of patients, I have only seen this once or twice. In those cases the person did not bother to wash his or her hands before testing and had used the same lancet over and over again. To avoid skin infections, wash your hands before testing and only use the same lancet once.

Another good reason to wash your hands in warm water before you test (especially if your hands are cold) is that there will be more blood close to the surface, and it will be easier to get a blood sample with only a small, gentle stab. If your hands are cold, then you may need to poke yourself harder and more than once before you can get enough blood for the test strip.

Where else can I test my blood glucose?

It is possible to prick the skin on a different part of your body. There are fewer nerve endings in the skin of your forearm, for example, and so pricking that skin is less painful. Places to prick your skin that are somewhere else (not your fingertips) are sometimes called "alternate sites."

Are glucose readings from alternate sites just as good as fingertip results?

No, they are not. To understand why pricking your finger will give you a more accurate blood glucose reading than using the skin of your forearm, you need to understand a little bit about how blood flows through your body.

The glucose level that matters is the glucose level in your arteries (the blood vessels that take blood from your heart to all the organs in your body). These arteries branch into smaller and smaller blood vessels that run through the tissue and organs in your body. The smallest blood vessels are called capillaries. As the capillaries pass through your liver, heart, brain, muscles, skin, and other organs, the cells in those organs take glucose and other nutrients out of the blood. The capillaries then connect to other blood vessels called veins. Blood flows back to your heart in your veins.

The amount of glucose in your veins will be lower than it is in your arteries. How much lower will depend on how much glucose was taken out by the cells in the organ that the blood passed through. If you are exercising vigorously, then the veins draining your muscles will have very low levels of glucose in them, because a lot was taken out by the muscles. When you prick your fingertip, you are testing capillary blood, and so the reading you get is very close to the level of glucose in your arteries. But when you test the skin on your forearm, this is mostly blood from your veins.

If you are fasting or resting for several hours, then the glucose level in your fingertip capillaries and forearm veins will be quite similar, so using the alternate site of the skin on your forearm is okay for a fasting blood glucose test. But if your blood glucose is rising fast (after a meal, for example), or is dropping fast (when you exercise or when your insulin is really "kicking in," for example), then the reading from your forearm skin will be quite misleading. It takes much longer for the glucose level in a forearm reading to change in these situations.

For example, if you have eaten a lot of carbohydrate, your fingertip glucose test will start rising in just a few minutes. By thirty minutes after the meal, it might be 100 mg/dL higher than it was before the meal. But thirty minutes after the meal, your forearm vein glucose will hardly have moved up at all. This can be even more of a problem if your blood glucose is falling. Let's say you have been exercising, and now you feel a bit sweaty, shaky, and anxious that your blood glucose might be dropping too low. If you check your blood glucose by testing from the skin of your forearm, you might get a reading that says your blood glucose is above 100 mg/dL (5.6 mmol/L), and so you might get false reassurance that your blood glucose is fine. But if you tested your fingertip blood glucose at the same time, it might give you a reading of under 60 mg/dL (3.3 mmol/L) which would tell you (correctly) that your blood glucose is too low and you should do something about it.

Why does my doctor tell me to check my blood glucose so often but then barely glances at the results?

I hope that this is not the case for you, but I have had many patients with diabetes complain that they go to a lot of bother to test themselves and record their blood glucose results to bring in to show their doctor, only to have the doctor ignore the results or pay very little attention to them. Maybe he or she was just tired that day or was behind schedule and in a rush. But if that happens more than once, you should ask your doctor what you are supposed to do with the results. As I said before, the main purpose for testing your blood glucose is so that you learn to interpret the results and understand why your numbers were high or low, but if you are having a hard time with this, your doctor should be able to help you. If he or she is not willing or able to do this for you, then you should consider changing to a doctor who can help you with this.

Does the fasting blood glucose need to be taken at the same time every day?

You don't have to test at exactly the same time every day, but your blood glucose is likely to be different at 9:00 a.m. than it was at 7:00 a.m., even if you have not eaten or exercised in between times. How much your fasting blood glucose changes in the morning depends a bit on what type of diabetes you have, whether you are taking insulin or pills for your diabetes, and what type of insulin or pills you take.

In the few hours before you wake up, your body pushes out hormones to help you get ready for the day ahead. Those hormones (corticosteroids and growth hormone, for example) make you more resistant to the effects of insulin and tend to drive your blood glucose up. If you have the time to do this, you might find it interesting to wake up and check your blood glucose every hour for two or three hours, without eating anything or taking insulin or pills and without exercising. This will give you a sense of how much your blood glucose changes. Many people get up a couple of hours later on the weekend than they do during the week, and so understanding how your blood glucose can change in the early morning can be helpful information to know.

What is a continuous glucose monitor?

Most people with diabetes hate pricking their finger and doing messy blood glucose tests. Some people hate it more than anything else about their diabetes. They long for the day when a machine will just tell them their blood glucose anytime they want, without having to think about it or prick their fingers. In the past few years, this dream has gotten a lot closer to reality. Several companies are finding ways to test the glucose level in the liquid under your skin.

The red cells in your blood float in liquid called plasma. A similar liquid, called interstitial fluid, can be found in the tissue under your skin. Sometimes this liquid comes to the surface as sweat. The glucose level in interstitial fluid is almost identical to the glucose level in your blood or plasma. One approach is to apply a device to the surface of the skin that passes a small electric current across the skin to open up your pores to allow interstitial fluid to come out into an absorbent pad, where it can be tested for glucose. One such device is the Glucowatch Biographer. You can find out more about it at www.glucowatch.com.

Two companies have got Federal Drug Administration (FDA) approval for their devices so far. When you attach this device you push a needle through the skin into the tissue underneath. There, a sensor checks the glucose level of the interstitial fluid every ten minutes. You can get more information at www.dexcom.com and www.medtronic.com. These devices are fairly expensive, both for the machine itself and for the sensors, which only last for a few days before they need to be replaced. However, if these types of devices become more reliable and more affordable, they offer exciting possibilities. They allow you to set an upper and lower blood glucose level, at which the device will warn you that your blood glucose is too high or too low. And even if your blood glucose is between those two levels, if it is falling fast, the machine can anticipate and warn you that you are dropping fast. In research trials on a few dozen people with type 1 diabetes, the subjects wearing one of these devices found that they had fewer high and low values, less hypoglycemia, and a lower HbA1c during several weeks of use.

Chapter 14

Interpreting Glucose Results

- Why should I test my blood glucose if I feel fine?
- How often should people with diabetes check their blood glucose?
- What is a normal blood glucose level for someone with diabetes?
- What blood glucose targets should I be aiming for?
- Why can I go to bed with a good blood glucose number, sleep all night, and wake up with a higher number?
- Why should I keep testing my blood glucose when the numbers don't make any sense?
- Why should I write the numbers down when the meter stores them all in its memory?
- What am I supposed to do with all the blood glucose information from my meter?
- Why can I eat the exact same thing two days in a row and get totally different blood glucose results afterward?
- Is it best to measure the blood glucose before or after a meal?
- How long after a meal should you test your blood glucose?
- What does it mean when my fasting blood glucose levels used to be good, and now they are higher—but I am not doing anything differently than I used to?

Why should I test my blood glucose if I feel fine?

Some people will "swear blind" to me that they can "tell" when their blood glucose is too high and when it is too low, and so they don't ever need to test their blood glucose. I know better than to argue with them. They are usually partly correct. Most people can tell when their blood glucose gets really low. I have already described the symptoms that you get with hypoglycemia (a low blood glucose), although the exact blood glucose level that triggers those symptoms varies a bit from one person to the next, but it is rare to feel hypoglycemic symptoms until the blood glucose is below 80 mg/dL (4.4 mmol/L). Most people can also tell when their blood glucose level gets really high. They feel thirsty and tired and have to go to the bathroom a lot. Again, people vary in how high the blood glucose needs to be before they notice it, but often it has to be over 300 mg/dL (16.7 mmol/L).

The problem is that, between those two extremes, most people cannot tell what their blood glucose is. You feel pretty much the same when your blood glucose is 110 mg/dL (6.1 mmol/L) as when it is 250 mg/dL (13.9 mmol/L). If you managed to keep your blood glucose around 200 mg/dL (11.1 mmol/L), you would probably feel fine for months on end, but that level of blood glucose will cause damage to your body. It is much healthier for you to keep your blood glucose average between 80–150 mg/dL (4.4–8.3 mmol/L), and the only way to do this is to check your blood glucose throughout the day.

Here is another way to think about it. If it was pitch black at night and you were asked to run through a dense forest of trees, you could make it to the other side. You could run until you slammed into a tree, pick yourself up, change direction, and run until you hit another tree, and eventually you would emerge out the other side with a few cuts, bruises, and bumps. But if you took a flashlight with you, you would get through the forest much faster and with fewer nasty surprises and injuries. A blood glucose monitor is a bit like having a flashlight to help with your diabetes. It lets you know when you are about to "hit" a problem due to a blood glucose surprise. It helps you to navigate through the forest of your life and avoid hitting too many trees.

How often should people with diabetes check their blood glucose?

I often hear doctors and nurses saying things like, "All diabetic patients should check their blood glucose level four times a day!" Sometimes they say "five times a day" or "seven times a day," perhaps "twice a day if you have type 2 diabetes, and four times a day if you have type 1 diabetes." I think that none of these statements is correct. For me, there is only one correct answer to that question. You should check your blood glucose as often as you think it is giving you useful information. After all, that is the only reason to test your blood glucose: so that you know what it is and can use that information to help you understand your diabetes better.

You may find that answer to be too vague or think that it puts too much responsibility onto you, so let me add a few things to think about. If you said to yourself, "Great. In that case, since I never get useful information from my blood glucose test, I should never test," then I think you need help to be able to interpret or understand your test results. And if you are someone who feels the need to test yourself twenty times a day, then I think you need guidance, too.

When you first get diabetes and start testing your blood glucose, it is hard to make sense of the results. Your doctor or nurse may ask you to test a few times a day, record the results, and then bring them back so that you can go over the results together. Your doctor or nurse may be able to help you understand the things that affect your blood glucose numbers and what causes them to go up and down. Some people find it much easier than others to figure out. Once you learn to use your blood glucose test results well, they can act like a very powerful flashlight guiding you through your life with diabetes.

What is a normal blood glucose level for someone with diabetes?

There is no single answer for this. Whether you have diabetes or not, a normal blood glucose varies throughout the day. The normal range for blood glucose when you wake, after you have had nothing to eat for eight to ten hours (a fasting blood glucose), is between 70–100 mg/dL (3.9–5.9 mmol/L). After a heavy meal, it might go up as high as 160 mg/dL (8.9 mmol/L), but it will never go above 200 mg/dL (11.1 mmol/L) if you do not have diabetes.

What blood glucose targets should I be aiming for?

You should try to get your blood glucose levels as close to the normal non-diabetic range as you can without ruining your life with too much hassle, expense, weight gain, or problems from low blood glucose (hypoglycemia). It is not easy getting your blood glucose close to normal. People vary in how much time, effort, and expense they are prepared or able to put into it. I have some patients with type 1 diabetes who manage to keep their HbA1c in the normal non-diabetic range (less than 6.0 percent), but it takes tremendous discipline and determination. Others feel that their lives are so stressful and complicated that they cannot cope with a complicated regimen. They have decided to accept a higher HbA1c because pushing it lower would ruin their quality of life. This can be a tricky decision. Although you may think that you can't get your HbA1c any lower, it may be that if you changed the type or dose of a pill or a shot of insulin, or if you changed something about your day-to-day life, it might become possible to get your HbA1c down safely. If you are over sixty, or if you are at higher than normal risk for cardiovascular disease (like heart attacks and strokes), then a target HbA1c of between 7 and 8 percent may be safer for you.

Why can I go to bed with a good blood glucose number, sleep all night, and wake up with a higher number?

This really baffles and frustrates a lot of people who have diabetes. Let's say you did everything right, ate just the right amount of healthy food, took the right amount of your pills or insulin, and went to bed feeling good about yourself with a blood glucose that was 130 mg/dL (7.2 mmol/L), say. You sleep all night and wake up with a blood glucose of 230 mg/dL (12.8 mmol/L). It doesn't seem possible unless you went sleepwalking and raided the refrigerator without knowing it! Where else did the extra glucose come from? It came from your own liver.

All human beings (whether or not we have diabetes) carry a store of glucose in our liver in the form of a kind of starch called glycogen. On average most people store about 200–300 grams of glycogen in their liver, which is equivalent to carrying about twenty slices of bread under your rib cage. We need this because we are warm-blooded mammals. Our brains and muscles need glucose, even when we are fasting or sleeping, so that they can keep working, so our liver trickles a steady amount of glucose into our bloodstream all night long. How much glucose is released and how fast it is released depends on how much insulin is around. If there is plenty of insulin in your system, then the liver does not convert glycogen to glucose, but if your insulin level is too low, or if your body does not respond to insulin as well as it should because you have insulin resistance, then your liver will pour glucose into your bloodstream all night long, causing a high blood glucose in the morning.

Why should I keep testing my blood glucose when the numbers don't make any sense?

You shouldn't, especially if the results don't help you to do anything differently. However, an experienced doctor or nurse should be able to help you. Here are some suggestions for you to try. Scan your page of confusing numbers and see if there are some that are close to the ideal range that you are hoping for. There may not be many, but if you can find some like that, ask yourself, "What did I do that day that worked so well?" Were you less stressed? Did you bring a packed lunch that day instead of eating out? Perhaps your meetings finished early, and you were able to go for a walk when you got home.

Even if you can't figure out exactly why a particular blood glucose number was close to the range you are hoping for, it is a good, positive exercise to go through to think of why you were successful. It is so easy for us to feel guilty and frustrated when we get a high blood glucose number. Try to stop thinking about blood glucose numbers as being "good" or "bad." The fact that your blood glucose was 436 mg/dL (24.2 mmol/L) doesn't mean that you are a "bad" person because that is a "bad" result. Perhaps you ate a large piece of cake an hour before taking that blood glucose test. That doesn't mean that you are a bad person. The best way to think about that result is to say to yourself, "Hmmm, that is a pretty convincing demonstration of how fast and how high my blood goes after I eat that much cake. Next time I should try having a smaller piece of cake or taking a bigger dose of insulin to cover it." With the right attitude, blood glucose testing can be incredibly helpful to you.

Why should I write the numbers down when the meter stores them all in its memory?

Call me old-fashioned if you like, but I don't think that modern "memory meters" are as "cool" as a lot of people do. Sure, it is possible to download them and have some clever piece of software print out pages upon pages of graphs and pie charts, but I am not impressed with how helpful the information is. You can end up drowning in data but not knowing what to do with it.

When used properly, the printouts can certainly show you patterns of how often you are too high or too low and what time of day you are most often in your target range. But I always worry when I ask people, "How are things going? Do you have particular concerns about your blood glucose levels?" and they just shrug, hand me the meter, and say, "Take a look; they are all in there!" That tells me that they are not getting useful information from blood glucose testing. They are not making connections between what the result was and what was going on in their life at the time to explain the result. I know it is a bother to write stuff down, but if you write down what you ate, how much insulin or how many pills you took, what was going on that day (in terms of stress or exercise or unusual events), then it makes it easier for you to look at it every day and make connections.

What am I supposed to do with all the blood glucose information from my meter?

There are three main reasons for checking your blood glucose level. The first is to look for overall patterns of when your blood glucose is running high or low. There can be a lot of variation in the blood glucose level at a particular time of day (like first thing in the morning, for example). But the weekly average of those numbers is a very stable and useful thing to look at. If the average level of blood glucose in the morning, taken over a one or two week period, shows that the blood glucose is too high, then it means that something needs to be changed in your treatment plan to improve the situation. The specific change will depend on the type of diabetes you have and what treatment you are taking.

In a similar way, if the blood glucose levels are always too low at lunchtime or too high at bedtime, this pattern will suggest specific changes that you can discuss with your diabetes health care team. The second reason to check your blood glucose is to make connections between how you feel or what you did and the blood glucose level. If you feel dizzy or sweaty or peculiar in some way, it is very helpful to check to see if your blood glucose at this time is too high or too low. If the blood glucose is normal when you feel peculiar, then it is likely that the symptoms are caused by something else. It can be useful to check your blood glucose one or two hours after eating a particular food or after doing a particular amount of exercise to see what effect it has on your blood glucose level.

The third reason to check your blood glucose is to use the information right then and there to make a change in a dose of diabetic medicine. Many people with type 1 diabetes will check their blood glucose before every meal. They will use the information to decide on what dose of fast-acting insulin to take to cover that meal. If the blood glucose is in a normal range (70–100 mg/dL, for example), they might take a certain dose of insulin, but if it was 101–140, they might take a higher dose. If it was even higher, they might take more insulin still. This variation in dose is sometimes called a *sliding scale* or a *pre-meal algorithm*.

Why can I eat the exact same thing two days in a row and get totally different blood glucose results afterward?

One of the hardest things to deal with when you have diabetes is learning to live with how unpredictable everything is. It is unfair that you can do the same things on two days and get different results. The problem is that there are lots of things that you do every day that are imprecise and that you have very little control over. Estimating how much food, especially carbohydrate, is in a meal takes practice and still gives you only an approximate idea. It is very hard to predict how much your stress will vary from day to day.

Even if you feel the same, there may be things going on in your subconscious that cause more stress on one day. Some days you are more active than others, running around at work or doing extra errands. And if you take insulin, this adds yet another level of uncertainty. You can give yourself exactly the same dose of insulin and inject it into the same part of your body (your abdomen, for example) on two different days, but the rate at which it gets absorbed into your bloodstream can vary quite a lot. And once you have injected that insulin, you can't take it back. It will not adjust itself just because your diet, stress, and activity have turned out differently than you expected that day.

Is it best to measure the blood glucose before or after a meal?

It depends what information you want to get. If you want to know how much fast-acting insulin to take before a meal, then checking your blood glucose immediately before the meal is a good idea. But if you want to check to see how high your blood glucose goes after eating a particular type of food, then testing after the meal makes sense. You may want to compare what happens to your blood glucose when you eat the same size of a piece of fruit or pie on two or three different days or at different times of the day. You may want to compare a small piece of pie one day with a larger piece another day. If you take fast-acting insulin before your meals, you might want to experiment by taking the same amount of food on several different days but varying how much insulin you take before the meal and comparing what happens to your blood glucose.

How long after a meal should you test your blood glucose?

How fast your blood glucose rises and how high it gets and how long it stays up after eating depends a lot on what it was that you ate. If you ate a jelly sandwich on white bread and washed it down with regular pop, your blood glucose would go up very quickly but would not stay high for long, so checking your blood glucose one hour after the meal would probably catch the peak. But if you ate a piece of pizza that was smothered in greasy meat and cheese, your blood glucose would go up more slowly and stay up longer, so the blood glucose two or even three hours after the meal would be higher than it was one hour after the meal. If you really want to know the overall effect of a particular meal on your blood glucose, you may need to check several times after the meal and do this on two or three different days.

What does it mean when my fasting blood glucose levels used to be good, and now they are higher—but I am not doing anything differently than I used to?

I often get asked to see people with diabetes because their doctor is frustrated with them and has labeled them as being "noncompliant." Let me say right here that I hate that term and try hard never to use it. It suggests that if these people had just done what their "perfect" doctor had told them to do (and so were "compliant"), then everything would have worked out perfectly! Very often when I talk to patients, it is clear that they are doing everything as "perfectly" as they can, and just as "perfectly" as they used to. But now it doesn't seem to be working. This is especially common for people with type 2 diabetes who used to wake up with fasting glucose levels in a good range (let's say 100–130 mg/dL, or 5.5–7.2 mmol/L), but over time their average keeps drifting up.

Now, no matter what they do, even if they eat almost nothing the night before, they can go to bed with a reasonable blood glucose but wake up with a really high number. What has happened, most likely, is that their body is gradually making less insulin than it used to. They used to make enough insulin to stop their liver from releasing too much glucose during the night, but now they don't make enough. Those patients are not "noncompliant." They just make less insulin than they used to, through no fault of their own, and so need an adjustment to the treatment that they take for their diabetes.

Chapter 15

Eating Right

- I'm not overweight, so why do I have diabetes?
- What is the best diet for someone with diabetes?
- What is a "balanced" diet?
- What are "empty" calories?
- Are all fats bad, or are some fats good for you?
- Does drinking too much alcohol cause diabetes?
- If I have diabetes, can I drink alcohol?
- Why does drinking alcohol make someone with diabetes more likely to have a low blood glucose (hypoglycemia)?
- Will drinking alcohol increase my risk of nerve damage?
- Is it true that there are health benefits from drinking alcohol?
- Is it best to use artificial sweeteners or real sugar in moderation?

I'm not overweight, so why do I have diabetes?

Two things need to happen for anyone to get diabetes. If you don't make enough insulin, then your body will not be able to keep your glucose level in the normal range. Type 2 diabetes is more common in people who are overweight because the extra weight makes your body resistant to the effects of insulin. Whether you get diabetes or not depends on how little insulin you make and how insulin-resistant you are. If you are normal weight but have developed diabetes, this means that your body doesn't make very much insulin at all. Although it is still possible that your diabetes might be able to be controlled by pills, it is more likely that you will need insulin shots to help keep your blood glucose close to normal.

What is the best diet for someone with diabetes?

First, let's go over the basics. There are three main types of food: protein, fat, and carbohydrate. Protein is essential to help us build strong bodies and muscles. We get protein from eating meat, fish, eggs, milk, cheese, and some vegetable proteins like soy beans (tempeh and tofu). We get fat from butter, margarine, oils, fatty meats, eggs, and in oily vegetables like avocadoes. Eating protein and fat will only cause your blood glucose to rise very slowly, because it takes your body several hours to break down the protein and fat and to turn it into glucose.

There are many different kinds of carbohydrates. Sugar, jams, honey, and fruit juices are examples of refined carbohydrate that is very quickly absorbed from your stomach and gut into your bloodstream. So when you eat refined carbohydrate, your blood glucose will rise very quickly. That is why these are good foods to eat if your blood glucose gets too low. All grains, bread, pasta, rice, and root crops like potatoes contain a lot of starch and carbohydrates that are less refined. Foods like lentils and beans contain unrefined carbohydrate with soluble fiber in it. When you eat this kind of carbohydrate, your blood glucose goes up much more slowly.

In the past few decades, nutritional research has shown quite consistent results. The kind of diet that will help reduce your risk of getting heart disease, high cholesterol, high blood pressure, or cancer is the same diet that helps prevent you from getting overweight. You should eat less fat (especially saturated fat), less protein (especially animal protein), and more unrefined carbohydrate (especially carbohydrate that is high in soluble fiber such as lentils and beans), grains, and fresh vegetables. Societies around the world that eat that kind of diet and combine it with an active lifestyle tend to have much lower rates of obesity, diabetes, and heart disease than countries like the United States, where we consume large amounts of fat, sugar, and protein processed into delicious, large portions that are sold fairly cheaply.

There may be some specific changes that you need to make in your diet, depending on what you are eating right now and what medical conditions you have, so it is a good idea to meet with a nutritionist or dietitian to get advice that is customized for you. But as a general rule, if you want to lose weight and stay healthy, you need to eat a balanced diet that contains fewer calories than you are burning up. Having said that, I know that it is easier said than done.

What is a "balanced" diet?

It means having a mixture of foods that includes vegetables, grains, fruits, vitamins, essential fats, and some protein. A "balanced" diet suggests that these things should be eaten in the right proportions every day, so it is not healthy to eat only meat for days on end or nothing but white bread and macaroni. If you grew up eating a healthy variety of food every day, you might find that you choose a healthy balance of foods quite naturally. But if you simply decide to eat whatever you feel like at every meal, you may find that you are eating too many high-fat, salty foods from fast-food restaurants and that you hardly ever eat fresh fruits and vegetables. The best way to know is to write down everything you eat for a few days and then look it over to see if there is a healthy variety of foods in there. If you can't tell, then ask to see a dietitian, and he or she can go over it with you. Developing healthy eating habits is an important way to stay healthy and keep your weight down.

What are "empty" calories?

As far as gaining weight is concerned, a calorie is a calorie. Whether the calorie comes from a healthy organic apple or from a spoonful of salty, processed macaroni and cheese with orange coloring, you will gain weight if the total number of calories you eat is more than the number you burn up from exercise and activity. What dietitians usually mean when they talk about "empty" calories are foods that contain no fiber or vitamins and have no other nutritional value. A group of dietitians would probably frown and wag their fingers at you if they saw you eating a piece of angel food cake with white frosting. You might hear whispers of "empty" calories. In truth, if you ate nothing but angel food cake with white frosting, that would not be healthy for you, because there is not a big enough variety of vitamins and other nutrients in it—but after several pieces, you would certainly not feel "empty"!

Are all fats bad, or are some fats good for you?

Not all fats are bad. Some fats are essential for a healthy diet. There are two things about fat that you should know. Fats are used by animals and plants to store energy. They are very calorie-dense. One teaspoonful of fat or oil contains almost as many calories as a tablespoonful of sugar or protein. So if you want to lose weight, you need to be careful not to eat too much fatty food. Fats also vary in how much they change the cholesterol and other fats (sometimes called lipids) in your blood. Saturated fats and trans fats are much more damaging to your arteries than unsaturated fats. In general, polyunsaturated and monounsaturated fats are healthier for us. Most vegetable oils are unsaturated. There seems to be extra benefit from monounsaturated fats (like olive oil), which is one of the reasons why a Mediterranean diet is so healthy.

Does drinking too much alcohol cause diabetes?

It can. Sometimes people who drink too much can get severe inflammation of their pancreas (called pancreatitis). If this happens over and over again, it can destroy enough of their pancreas that they no longer make enough insulin to keep their blood glucose normal. This is one of the causes of secondary diabetes.

If I have diabetes, can I drink alcohol?

Yes, you can, but there are things to think about. First, alcohol contains quite a lot of calories (seven calories for every gram, which is more than protein or carbohydrate and almost as many calories per gram as fat). So if you drink regularly, it will be harder to lose weight. Besides, many people eat while they drink. Alcohol can increase your appetite. If you are acting oddly because your blood glucose is too low and someone smells alcohol on your breath, they may assume that you are drunk and so not give you the help you need. Even modest amounts of alcohol can increase your risk of hypoglycemia, and if you drink to excess, it makes you much more likely to get nerve damage.

Why does drinking alcohol make someone with diabetes more likely to have a low blood glucose (hypoglycemia)?

When your blood glucose gets too low, your brain sends signals to your body to push out hormones that "tell" your liver to release glucose into your blood to bring your blood glucose up again.

Alcohol interferes with those signals and makes it harder for glucose to be released from your liver. This can happen even if you have only drunk a moderate amount of alcohol. I see this most often with healthy, young college students who have type 1 diabetes. They spend a couple of hours playing basketball or soccer and then have a couple of beers at the end of the evening. They may even have food along with the beer and check their blood glucose before they go to bed and find that it is fine. But then they are found unconscious or thrashing about or having a seizure in the middle of the night.

There are two factors causing this situation. After prolonged and vigorous exercise, your muscles get emptied of all of their stored glucose. So for several hours after you stop exercising, your muscles continue to suck glucose out of the blood to refill their stores. That causes the blood glucose to keep dropping. You should be able to release glucose from your liver to keep the blood glucose higher, but the alcohol in your system makes this much harder. Because of this, your blood glucose can drop to dangerous levels. One other factor is that if you drink enough alcohol to make your thinking fuzzy, you may be less able to tell that your blood glucose is dropping too low, even if you are still awake.

Will drinking alcohol increase my risk of nerve damage?

It will if you drink too much. Alcohol is a drug that is toxic to the nerves. Even people who do not have diabetes can get quite severe neuropathy if they drink too much alcohol. The combination of poorly controlled diabetes and too much alcohol can make painful neuropathy much more likely.

Is it true that there are health benefits from drinking alcohol?

Yes. A number of studies in the past few years have shown that drinking up to two alcoholic drinks per day for men and up to one alcoholic drink per day for women may reduce your risk of heart disease. The original studies said that this benefit was from drinking red wine, but more recent studies show that modest amounts of any alcoholic drink provide some benefit. Now, don't misinterpret this. I am not suggesting that you should start drinking if you have never drunk alcohol in your life or if you purposely avoid drinking it for other reasons. In those studies, people who drink no alcohol have quite good outcomes, and people who drink to excess do much worse. But it is interesting that a moderate amount of alcohol might actually be good for you.

Is it best to use artificial sweeteners or real sugar in moderation?

Unless your blood glucose is low and you want to bring it up fast to avoid hypoglycemia, it is best to drink liquids that are sugar-free. Whether you drink plain water or flavored drinks sweetened with artificial sweeteners is up to you and how you like things to taste. Some people dislike the taste of artificial sweeteners so much that they would rather drink water. Other people avoid artificial sweeteners, because they believe that these are bad for you and can damage your body. There are many urban legends going round and round on the internet about diseases "caused" by Nutrasweet or other sweeteners. I have not seen any reputable scientific studies linking the use of artificial sweeteners and any weird illnesses or symptoms. While it is probably not a great idea to drink gallons of diet pop every day, they are fine to drink in moderation.

Chapter 16

Losing Weight

- Why do I gain weight no matter what I eat?
- If I lose weight, will my diabetes go away?
- Why is it that the more I try to get my blood glucose levels down, the more I gain weight?
- I've lost weight lots of times on all sorts of different diets, but then I regain it again. How can I keep the weight off?
- Why is "portion control" so important, and what is a "portion" anyway?
- What are the best diet pills to use to help you lose weight?
- What is bariatric surgery?
- When is bariatric surgery a good idea?

Why do I gain weight no matter what I eat?

I know that it can often seem that no matter what you eat, you still gain weight. But the hard fact is that the only way you can gain weight over time is if you take in more calories than your body is burning up. Some people can gain weight by holding on to fluid, and if you think that is your problem, then you need to see your doctor to figure out how to prevent that. But most people gain weight because they are adding fat.

If you are gaining fat, then you are eating more calories than you are using up every day. We get calories from the food we eat. Every gram of carbohydrate or protein gives us about 4 calories; every gram of fat gives us 9 calories; and every gram of alcohol gives us 7 calories. It doesn't matter where the calories come from. If you take in 2,000 calories every day but only burn up 1,900 calories every day, then over time, that extra 100 calories will be stored as fat in your body, and you will gain weight. How do you "burn up" calories? You use them to give your muscles fuel to move around, to keep your body warm, to supply your heart and brain and all of your other organs with energy to stay healthy. So why does it seem as though you can gain weight no matter what you eat? There are a couple of common reasons.

As we get older, our metabolism changes. I remember when I was in my teens, I would come home from school and eat half a loaf of bread with jam and cheese on it (a rough estimate of about 1,000 calories!) and then have a full three-course meal about an hour later. Yet I never gained weight back then. If I ate like that nowadays, I would double in size in six months! As a teenager, I was growing in height and had a very active lifestyle. Now that I am fully grown, my body needs fewer calories. I have less time to exercise, and I need to exercise more carefully and slowly, because I have more stiffness and aches and pains than I used to. Because of that, I need to consciously eat less. I need to pay attention.

You may think that you are not eating very much, but if you are gaining weight, you are probably eating more than you think. Maybe you are taking bigger portions of food than you used to; maybe you hardly notice when you "graze" on snacks; or maybe you have started having an extra cocktail or glass of wine with your evening meal. Whatever it is, you must be sneaking extra calories into your mouth if you are gaining weight. Many people find that if they start keeping a diary and writing down every single thing they eat during the day, it becomes clear where those extra calories are coming from.

If I lose weight, will my diabetes go away?

It depends on what type of diabetes you have. If you have type 1 diabetes and don't make any insulin, then no amount of weight loss will make your diabetes go away. In fact, it would be very dangerous for you to try to lose weight and stop taking your insulin. If you have type 2 diabetes and still make quite a lot of insulin, it is possible that—if you change your diet and lose weight—you will become a lot less resistant to insulin, so that the amount of insulin your body makes becomes enough to keep your blood glucose levels normal again. This happens to women who get diabetes during pregnancy (which is called gestational diabetes). Once they deliver the baby and lose all the weight that they gained during the pregnancy, then their diabetes goes away again.

I have seen people who were able to come off insulin or stop taking their diabetes pills when they managed to change their lifestyle so that they ate less, exercised regularly, and lost weight. And even if your diabetes doesn't go away completely, it is likely to be much easier to keep your blood glucose levels closer to normal when you lose weight.

Why is it that the more I try to get my blood glucose levels down, the more I gain weight?

There are a couple of reasons why this happens, and it depends a bit on what type of diabetes you have and what treatment you are on. Let's say your blood glucose levels are running over 200 mg/dL (11.1 mmol/L) most of the time and your HbA1c is over 9.0 percent. Your kidneys will filter out a lot of that extra sugar, and you flush it down the toilet. You could be losing 500 calories a day or more in your urine. If you make changes to your diabetes treatment by increasing the dose of pills or insulin to bring your blood glucose level down, but you don't change what you are eating, you will no longer lose those extra calories down the toilet. As a result, you gain weight.

Also, if your diabetes has been out of control for several weeks you will feel hungrier and may have started eating more without realizing it. Again, when you make changes to improve your blood glucose levels but don't change your eating habits, then you will gain weight. If the treatment you take for your diabetes causes a higher insulin level in your body during the day and between meals, this will make you hungrier and at more risk of a low blood glucose level (hypoglycemia), and so you may eat extra food to compensate. Drugs that stimulate insulin release (like sulfonylureas and meglitinides) and insulin itself can make you feel hungry or hypoglycemic between meals.

The best way to avoid weight gain when you make changes to improve your blood glucose level is to be conscious about what you are eating. It often helps to write down what you eat. You can also ask your doctor to help choose the best type of pill or insulin to make weight gain less likely.

I've lost weight lots of times on all sorts of different diets, but then I regain it again. How can I keep the weight off?

I have had patients say to me, "You know, in all the diets I have tried over all these years, I have lost my entire body weight two times over, and yet here I am today, heavier than I have ever been." The problem is that most diets feel like a punishment. You make yourself eat less by force of willpower, because you know it is for your own good. And the more weight you lose, the more your body sends your brain signals that it is hungry. At some point you decide to give yourself a break from your diet, and so you regain the weight. Long-term studies have followed people who go on weight-reducing diets, and five years later, less than 10 percent of those people have kept the weight off.

Some people are able to keep the weight off permanently, however. There are three things that those people tend to do that help them to keep their weight off. They change their lifestyle in a permanent way so that they get regular exercise almost every day. An ideal amount of exercise for most people to get is about thirty minutes at least five days a week. They continue to write down what they eat every day so that they are always conscious of what they are eating. They stay connected with a support group of other people who are trying to maintain weight loss. Instead of eating or drinking when they get stressed, they find other ways to reduce stress without adding calories. It is only when you can permanently change your eating and exercise habits that you can keep your weight at a healthier level.

Why is "portion control" so important, and what is a "portion" anyway?

The size of a "normal portion" has been steadily increasing in the United States. The food industry wants us to eat bigger amounts so that they can sell us more food. If you compare the size of plates and the amount that was put on them at mealtimes in the 1950s to what we are served now, it is amazing to see the changes.

One of the keys to successful management of your weight and of your diabetes is to be conscious of how much you are eating from day to day. Dietitians can be very helpful in coaching you on how to do this. Some of them use a technique called the "Idaho Plate Method." You can find out more about that at http://platemethod.com/.

Another simple approach is to use your own hands as a guide. A healthy portion of meat for you to eat at a meal is a piece that is the size of the palm of your hand. A medium potato or apple is about the size of your closed fist. Obviously bigger people tend to have bigger hands and fists, but since they probably need bigger portions, then this simple approach usually helps quite a bit.

What are the best diet pills to use to help you lose weight?

I'm afraid that the answer is "none of them." Everyone would like weight loss to be easy. If we could just eat a pill that would stop us feeling hungry or would prevent us from absorbing those calories, then it would be much easier to lose weight. Drugs are available that will do both of those things, but the long-term results from clinical research trials are very disappointing. Most of the drugs that suppress our appetite are derived from amphetamine drugs. They change the chemical signals inside our brain to make us feel less hungry. For the first few months of using them, they can seem to be miraculously effective.

Drugs like fenfluramine and phentermine (which were often given together as "fen-phen") or dexfenfluramine (which was marketed as Redux) were incredibly popular a few years ago. There are two big problems with these drugs. First, the effect did not last very long. People usually had lost most of the weight they were going to lose by six months, but by a year, they had begun to regain some of it. By two years, they had regained even more. The even bigger problem with these drugs is that they have significant side effects. If you use them for years and years, they can increase the pressure in the blood vessels in your lungs (a condition called pulmonary hypertension). They can also damage the valves in your heart. Those are very serious side effects for drugs that do so little long-term good. These drugs clearly were doing more harm than good, and so they were taken off the market.

Another drug that has been used to help people lose weight is orlistat (Xenical). This drug blocks the enzyme in your guts that helps you digest and absorb fat (an enzyme called lipase). So if you take orlistat, you will not be able to absorb so much fat, and you will flush those calories down the toilet instead of absorbing them into your body, where they would be put into your own fat deposits. It sounds great, and it does work for a while. But once again, most people have lost most of their weight by six to twelve months and are beginning to regain their weight by eighteen to twenty-four months after the start. There are lots of reasons for this. The side effects from orlistat are a bit unpleasant. You have loose bowel movements, and they smell bad. And the more weight you lose, the hungrier you tend to feel. Some people start to figure out that if they eat less fat but more carbohydrate and protein in their diet, then they feel better. They also start gaining more weight again, because the orlistat doesn't prevent you from absorbing carbs and protein.

As you can imagine, there are a lot of drug companies doing research to find other "weight loss drugs." Maybe someday it will be much easier to lose weight, but for now, I am not impressed with how well they help people. If you are hoping for results that will be permanent (or at least keep your weight down for several years), then weight loss drugs are not the answer.

What is bariatric surgery?

Bariatric surgery refers to the various surgical procedures performed to treat obesity. One approach is to put a band round the lower end of the tube that leads from your mouth to your stomach (which is called the esophagus). Another is to stitch up part of the stomach to make it smaller, or to disconnect part of your guts and reconnect it to make your guts shorter. This is sometimes called gastric bypass surgery. Combinations of those procedures are done quite commonly nowadays to help with weight loss.

Why do they work? We don't know all the reasons. If the stomach is smaller, maybe you feel full after eating just a small amount. If the length of your gut is smaller, you absorb less food. It turns out that there is another reason, too. Your stomach makes a hormone called ghrelin. This hormone tells your brain that you are hungry. When you lose weight by dieting, your ghrelin levels go up, and so your brain feels hungrier and hungrier. But after some forms of gastric bypass surgery, the ghrelin levels go down, even after you lose a lot of weight. Those people do not feel nearly so hungry, and so it is easier for them to keep their weight off.

I don't think this is a perfect solution for everyone who is overweight. It is a major surgical operation with quite a few side effects and complications. Although it is rare, some people die as a result of the surgery. But for some people, it can have dramatic and life-changing benefits.

When is bariatric surgery a good idea?

The people who I usually refer for bariatric surgery have a body mass index of over 40 kg/m2. They are people who are really motivated and have tried many times to really work on improving their eating habits. They are sensible folk who are stable psychologically, as far as I can tell. Their diabetes is not well controlled, despite high doses of several medicines and insulin. They have other complications as a result of their diabetes and their weight. Often they have high blood pressure (hypertension) and high cholesterol and triglyceride levels. Some of them have sleep apnea. I make sure that I send them to a surgeon who does a lot of this kind of surgery and gets really good results.

Bariatric surgery is not for everyone. Some insurance companies "cover it" under certain circumstances, but others do not. If you are considering it, you should investigate the insurance options further or ask what it would cost if you had to pay for it yourself.

Chapter 17

CARBOHYDRATE COUNTING

- What is the glycemic index?
- Why do dietitians want me to eat more carbohydrates than I want to?
- What is carbohydrate counting?
- Why do I need to look at all carbohydrates and not just sugar?
- Why are most doctors so down on low carb diets like the Atkins diet?
- What are "net carbs"?
- What is the best way to use carb counting?

What is the glycemic index?

Not all types of carbohydrate have the same effect on your blood glucose. They have different numbers of small building blocks (or sugar molecules) stuck together. Simple carbohydrates have only one or two sugar molecules stuck together. Glucose has just one. Table sugar has two. Complex carbohydrates like starches (potatoes, rice, flour, bread, pasta) have many hundreds of sugar molecules stuck together.

For many years it was assumed that complex carbohydrates would be broken down much more slowly than simple sugars, and so the blood glucose would rise more slowly after eating starches than after eating table sugar or fruit juice or jam. It was also assumed that carbohydrates that contained a lot of fiber (like brown rice or whole wheat bread) would be absorbed more slowly than white rice and white bread. A series of research studies on this topic in the 1970s and 1980s showed that these assumptions may not always be true.

The researchers fed people 50 grams of different kinds of carbohydrate and measured how quickly their blood glucose went up, how high it got, and how quickly it came back down again. They found that eating 50 grams of table sugar and 50 grams of white bread gave an almost identical profile. In both cases the blood glucose went up very quickly, had a high peak, and came down again quickly after the food had all been absorbed. They called that response a high glycemic index and gave it a value of 100.

Then they compared the response that people had to other foods and to white bread. If something was absorbed even faster and had a higher peak than white bread or table sugar, then it would have a glycemic index of over 100. But if something was absorbed more slowly and with a lower peak, it would have a glycemic index of under 100. To their surprise, they found that whole wheat bread and brown rice were absorbed just about as fast as white bread (with glycemic indices of 96–99); but white rice had a lower glycemic index (83), and white spaghetti was even lower (66). The popular breakfast cereal cornflakes had an even higher glycemic index than white bread (119), whereas ice cream had a very low glycemic index (49)!

This does not mean that you should eat ice cream for breakfast rather than cornflakes, however. It does show us that how quickly we absorb our food is more complicated than we used to think. Because it is sometimes surprising what effect certain foods will have on your blood glucose, it is a good idea to check your blood glucose before you eat a new type of food, and then test again one or two hours afterward to see how high your blood glucose goes and how long it stays up. This is particularly important for foods that you like to eat fairly often.

In general if you eat foods with a low glycemic index, your blood glucose will not rise so high after a meal, and that makes it easier to control the swings in blood glucose that occur after meals. But if you are feeling as though your blood glucose is dropping too low (hypoglycemia), then you want to eat a food with a high glycemic index (like fruit juice, table sugar, or white bread). Half a can of tinned soy beans is not going to help you much if you are about to pass out from hypoglycemia!

Why do dietitians want me to eat more carbohydrates than I want to?

Most dietitians will tell you that 50–60 percent of your calories should come from complex carbohydrates (especially those with soluble fiber and low glycemic indices) and that you should spread it out throughout the day (with 45–60 grams of carbohydrate at most meals and 15–30 grams of carbohydrate in snacks in between meals). They often advise you to take some protein along with the carbohydrate to help slow the absorption.

There are a couple of good reasons why they give you that advice. A diet high in carbohydrate that is slowly absorbed and contains only modest amounts of healthy protein and fat has been shown to be good for you in the long term. Spreading the carbohydrate out during the day helps prevent you from feeling hungry and then overeating. People who try to eat almost nothing during the day in order to lose weight usually are not successful. Often they feel so ravenous when they come home at night that they overeat in the evening.

Depending on the type of pills or insulin that you take for your diabetes, it can be important to take enough carbohydrate throughout the day to prevent your blood glucose dropping too low and causing hypoglycemia. That is not quite as important as it used to be, however. I used to hear people with diabetes complain that they felt they had to overeat on carbohydrates to "feed their insulin peak." Because of that, they gained weight. A better solution for that problem is to change to a different type of insulin or pill that does not force the insulin level to be so high between meals. Most dietitians will take time to listen to you and to give you advice that is tailored to your lifestyle, so it is usually well worth your while spending time with one.

What is carbohydrate counting?

Because it is carbohydrate foods that have the biggest effect on your blood glucose, it is important to pay attention to the amount of carbohydrate that you are eating at a meal. Even if you don't use insulin, it is a good idea to learn to estimate how much carbohydrate you are eating. A dietitian can give you a lot of help. There are also a lot of books and websites out there that go into this in detail. The American Diabetes Association has very useful information that does not have commercial bias, http://www.diabetes.org/for-parents-and-kids/diabetes-care/carb-count.jsp. There are books and websites that tell you how many grams of carbohydrate are contained in many popular foods. One that many of my patients like is called Calorie King (http://www.calorieking.com/).

There are different ways to do carbohydrate counting. You may have been taught to think in term of "carbohydrate exchanges," which counts carbohydrate in 15 gram portions. So a typical thin slice of bread is about 15 grams, or "one carb portion"; a sandwich contains 30 grams, or two portions, and so on. Most foods now contain a label that tells you what they contain. You should look for where it says "total carbohydrates."

You also need to check the label to find out how many "servings per container" there are. Consider two cans of soup. The cans are the same brand and the same size. The chicken noodle soup contains 11 grams per serving, while the tortilla soup contains 27 grams per serving. Both cans contain two servings per container. So if I ate the whole can of tortilla soup, I would get 54 grams of carbohydrate, but the whole can of chicken noodle soup contains less than half of that at 22 grams. If you are used to thinking in terms of 15-gram carb portions, you will have to "round up" to the nearest portion. So if you want to eat three carb portions (or 45 grams) for lunch, you could make a sandwich with two slices of bread along with about a third of a can of the tortilla soup; but to get the same amount of carbohydrate, you would need to eat about three-quarters of the can of chicken noodle soup along with your sandwich.

Why do I need to look at all carbohydrates and not just sugar?

Even if you have diabetes, your body is incredibly good at breaking down complex, starchy carbohydrates into molecules of glucose that are then absorbed into your bloodstream. Your blood glucose will rise just about as fast after eating a piece of bread or a spoonful of sugar or mashed potatoes. How high your blood glucose goes after a meal depends, to some extent, on the type of carbohydrate and what else you ate along with it. But the overall amount of carbohydrate is by far the most important thing to track. A lot of people underestimate how much carbohydrate they are eating and get a big surprise when they check their blood glucose after a meal. So although you may find it interesting to look at the amount of fiber or sugar that something contains when you check food labels, the most important thing that will affect how high your blood glucose goes after a meal is the total amount of carbohydrate in your meal.

Why are most doctors so down on low carb diets like the Atkins diet?

High protein/low carb diets like the Atkins diet "work" because they are carbohydrate deficient diets. Since your body needs carbohydrate (your brain can't function without using glucose as its fuel), when you eat a low carb diet, your body has to turn some of the protein and fat that you ate into glucose. This is a slow process and one that uses up a lot of energy. As part of the chemical reactions that occur in your body to convert fat and protein to glucose, you produce acid and become a little dehydrated. Many people are delighted at how quickly they lose weight when they start a low carb diet, but most of the early weight loss is from dehydration. Many people feel a little nauseated when they start a low carb diet, and so they don't feel like eating as much. A combination of all of those things does make a low carb diet an effective way to lose weight.

Several well-designed clinical trials have compared weight loss using a low carb diet with a low calorie diet that is more balanced with carbohydrate, protein, and fat. In all cases, the people on low carb diets got slightly more weight loss and lost it quicker than those on the other diets. Although doctors worried that the low carb diets might lead to higher cholesterol levels or higher blood pressure, that was not found in these studies. So why are so many doctors still "down" on low carb diets? It is because we do not know how healthy these diets are when someone eats like that for years and years.

No studies have shown that people are better at keeping their weight off with low carb diets than with any other kind of diet. It may be several more years before we know the long-term effects of diets that are high in fat and protein and really low in carbohydrate. My feeling is that they are not harmful to try in the short term, especially if you eat healthier types of protein and fat. But in the long term, I am quite sure that a diet that is high in grains, unrefined carbohydrates like lentils and beans, and relatively low in protein and fat will be healthier for your body.

What are "net carbs"?

This term is used by people who are pushing low carb diets. They take the total amount of carbohydrate and then subtract the amount of fiber and call the result *net carbs*. It makes it sound as though there is less carbohydrate in what you are eating, but there isn't. The fact that there is fiber in the food sometimes means that it will be absorbed more slowly but sometimes has very little effect. And even if the fiber does slow down the absorption of the carbohydrate, you still end up absorbing all of the carbohydrate eventually.

I think the term net carbs is very misleading. Some of my patients who are getting tired of their low carb diets are delighted to tell me that they have found "low carb bread." This is quite ridiculous, since bread is almost 100 percent carbohydrate. The only way to eat a slice of bread that contains less carbohydrate is to eat a smaller or thinner slice! Subtracting the grams of fiber does not magically make the carbs disappear. If you want to keep track of how much carbohydrate you are eating, stick to counting "total carbohydrates" on food labels.

What is the best way to use carb counting?

It depends on what type of diabetes you have and how much time and effort you want to put into it. If you are frustrated with how much your blood glucose levels swing around from day to day, it is a good idea to learn to do carbohydrate counting and then keep a diary for a few days of exactly how much carbohydrate you eat at the same times on different days. You may be very surprised to see how variable your eating patterns are. Your blood glucose results might start making a lot more sense and might be less variable if you worked on eating a similar carbohydrate profile from day to day.

For example you may be someone who doesn't like to eat a lot in the morning. You might decide that just 30 grams of carbohydrate is enough for breakfast, 15 grams for a mid-morning snack, 45 grams at lunch, and 90 grams with your evening meal. If you ate that same "carbohydrate profile" every day and adjusted your diabetic medicines to work well with that, then your blood glucose results are likely to become less variable and unpredictable. Some people do not like to eat the same amounts at the same times every day. Maybe you prefer to vary what you have for lunch. If you learn to count carbohydrate, you will be more aware of when you are about to have a meal that has less or more carbohydrate than you usually eat. You can then adjust how much exercise you do or how much insulin you give to help deal with the carbohydrate.

For people who use a dose of fast-acting insulin before every meal, it is possible to make quite sophisticated calculations using carbohydrate counting. Most of us are more insulin resistant in the morning than we are later in the day. You may need more insulin to cover carbohydrate in the morning than for the same amount of carbohydrate in the afternoon or evening. I have a patient with type 1 diabetes who calculates the amount of carbohydrate that she is about to eat at every meal. At breakfast she takes 1 unit of fast-acting insulin to cover every 7.5 grams of carbohydrate; but at lunch she takes 1 unit for every 10 grams of carbohydrate, and at her evening meal she only needs 1 unit to cover every 15 grams.

Chapter 18

HEALTHY EXERCISE

- Why do I have to exercise if I don't enjoy it?
- How can I get past my excuses not to exercise?
- Why should I exercise if I feel worse afterward?
- Is it safe for someone with diabetes to exercise?
- Should I get an EKG and other fancy tests before I start an exercise program?
- How often should I test my blood glucose if I am going to exercise?
- What is a pedometer, and how do you use one?
- What should I look for when choosing a pedometer?
- How can I exercise safely without developing a low blood glucose (hypoglycemia)?
- Why does exercise have a bigger effect on my blood glucose in the afternoon than it does in the morning?
- Why does my blood glucose sometimes drop several hours after I have finished exercising?
- Why does my blood glucose sometimes go up instead of down after exercise?

Why do I have to exercise if I don't enjoy it?

You don't. Like so many things about how you go about your life, you have choices. And although doctors or nurses might "prescribe" an exercise program for you, it is up to you if you do it. You can choose whether to take your pills or insulin shots or how often to prick your finger to check your blood glucose. The same thing is true for exercise. You have to decide for yourself that it is somehow worth it for your overall health and happiness. Then you need to find ways to overcome all the barriers that prevent you from exercising. The benefits of exercise are easy to list. It is a long list. Exercise is good for your heart, helps lower blood pressure, protects you against bone thinning (osteoporosis), improves your mood, and helps depression. When you exercise regularly, you become more responsive to insulin, so all your pills and insulin work better. It helps lower your blood glucose and makes it easier to keep weight off.

So if exercise is so incredibly worthwhile, why is it so hard for many of us? The list of excuses that we all make for ourselves is even longer than the list of benefits. We don't have time. We don't enjoy it. We are embarrassed at how we look. We don't think we can do enough to make any difference. There's no room to exercise at home. The weather is too bad for exercise outside (that's an easy one to use if, like me, you grew up in Scotland and now live in the Pacific Northwest). The gym is too far away or too expensive. It is boring. We don't have anyone to do it with.

How can I get past my excuses not to exercise?

You can make a list of all the benefits you will get if you exercise. You can write down some possible ways to overcome your barriers. Then you can choose one of those and come up with a specific thing you could do today to get yourself going. In other words you can take concrete, do-able "baby steps" toward your goal. Remember, any amount of exercise is better than none. Even if it seems too hard to do thirty minutes of exercise every day, start with less time and build up gradually. The key thing is to start to do some exercise every day so that it becomes part of your daily routine.

There are many helpful books written that give more detailed ways to change your behavior for the better. One that my patients like is *101 Tips for Behavior Change* by Robert Anderson, Martha Funnell, and colleagues. You can check it out online. The American Diabetes Association has an extensive library of practical books for people with diabetes (www.diabetes.org). Websites that are focused on practical ways to help you get started with walking programs in your community include WalkAmerica (www.walkamerica.org) and America on the Move (www.americaonthemove.org).

Why should I exercise if I feel worse afterward?

You shouldn't. You should talk to your doctor about this. The advice you will get will depend on how bad you feel. If you are getting chest pain or feel dizzy, breathless, nauseated, or weak, then you should not be exercising until you get a medical examination and some tests to figure out what is going on. If the problem is that you feel stiff or your muscles or joints ache afterward, then the solution might be as simple as wearing shoes with more cushioning or doing some stretching before you start. You need to use your own judgment. If you start exercise slowly and build it up gradually over time, you should feel better and better afterward. If you don't, then ask your doctor for help. Don't give up.

Is it safe for someone with diabetes to exercise?

Everyone is different. How safe exercise is depends on how old you are, how fit you are, how long you have had diabetes, and what other medical problems you have. For many people, simply starting to add some moderate exercise to your daily routine is perfectly safe. "Moderate exercise" means exercise that is enough to raise your heart rate but still allows you to carry on a conversation. Brisk walking with a friend is a good example. Starting with fifteen minutes a day and building up to at least thirty minutes every day is a great goal. If you do not feel good when you exercise, you should stop and go see your doctor.

Should I get an EKG and other fancy tests before I start an exercise program?

Calling something an "exercise program" makes it seem more grand and important than it really is. Exercise is a very natural activity for animals like us and is something that we should all try to include as part of everyday life. Whether you need an electrical tracing of your heart (an electrocardiogram, or EKG or ECG) or a treadmill test or other tests is up to your doctor. If you feel as if you are out of shape and have not exercised for a long time, and if you are planning to start a "program" that will be a lot of exercise, then getting a medical check up before you start is a good idea.

How often should I test my blood glucose if I am going to exercise?

Checking your blood glucose before, during, and after exercise can give you a lot of useful information. Exactly how often you test depends on how long you are exercising and how vigorously you exercise. Here are some of the things to consider. If you do the same amount of exercise at the same time every day, the changes in your blood glucose will be quite similar, but if you exercise in the morning on one day and in the evening on another day, it affects your blood glucose differently. If you exercise when your blood glucose is high (over 250 mg/dL or 13.9 mmol/L, for example), you may find you get tired, don't get a good workout, and your blood glucose is higher afterward instead of lower.

If you plan to do a particular kind of exercise for a certain length of time on a regular basis (like thirty minutes of swimming in the morning three times a week or forty minutes of walking every day after dinner), it is a good idea to test your blood glucose before you start, as soon as you finish, and then an hour or two later. If you do this on a few different days, you should see a pattern. If you are exercising for longer than thirty minutes, especially if it is vigorous exercise like cycling or soccer or basketball, you should test every fifteen minutes during the exercise as well as afterward. You can see how low your blood glucose drops and can experiment with taking different amounts of food before or during the exercise the next time to see what effect that has.

What is a pedometer, and how do you use one?

Pedometers have become popular in the past few years for good reasons. They are small gadgets that are lighter than a cell phone and can be clipped to your waistband. Inside, they have a moving switch (like a seesaw or teeter-totter) that "counts" every time you take a step. So if you go for a walk around the block or to the store and back, it will tell you how many steps you took.

The reason why I like them is because they give you something positive to work toward. When you have diabetes, you are always being told what you should not do! "Don't eat cakes or candy. Don't ever walk barefoot. Don't...don't...don't." But with a pedometer, you have something you can do—and the more you do, the better. I'm sure when you see a high number on your blood glucose meter, you don't like it because it means that you ate too much or were stressed or took too little insulin or something like that. But on a pedometer, the higher the number is the happier you will be, because it means you have walked farther and done more exercise.

Here is a good way to start using a pedometer. Every morning, reset it to zero and then just go about your regular daily life. Every night when you go to bed, record how many steps you took that day. You can record it in the same book where you write down your blood glucose readings, your insulin doses, and the amounts of carbohydrate that you ate. At the end of the week, you can take the average (by adding all the pedometer numbers and dividing by seven). You might also notice patterns. Let's say at the end of the week, you averaged 3,400 steps per day. But maybe you notice that on one of these days you had 5,100 steps. What was different that day? Did you miss your bus stop and have to walk five extra blocks out of your way? Did you go for a walk with a friend over lunch?

A pedometer just makes you more conscious about what you are doing and how much activity you have in your daily life. It makes it easy for you to set goals to be more active. If you try to add a thousand steps every day, you will be well on your way to adding regular exercise to your life. Start using the stairs instead of the elevator. Park farther away from the mall or from your office. Go for a walk over lunch or in the evening. When you take the dog for a walk, go three extra blocks before turning for home. You will be amazed at how easy it is to gradually add steps to your daily routine. If adding a thousand steps per day gets too easy, then go for adding two thousand or three thousand. If you can gradually increase the number of steps you take every day, and you can maintain that for several weeks, you will begin to see and feel the benefit in your mood, energy level, blood glucose average, blood pressure, and weight.

You hear a lot about ten thousand steps being a kind of magic number for using a pedometer. A lot of people think that if you can get yourself up to doing ten thousand steps per day, then you will be able to lose weight and keep it off. You will also get a lot of heart benefit when you are up to that level of daily activity. It is certainly a good goal to shoot for, but if you find you just can't do that much, do not get discouraged. Any amount of activity and exercise is better than none. Build up to a goal that you can keep doing for months or years on end, and only increase it when you feel that you can do it comfortably.

What should I look for when choosing a pedometer?

Pedometers are affordable, starting at ten to twenty dollars. They have buttons to set the time, enter your weight, reset the counter, and so forth. Some of them have the buttons exposed on the outside. I prefer the kind that has a cover that protects the buttons (it can be annoying to bump into a desk in the afternoon and have your pedometer reset to zero by mistake!). Some pedometers have extras like FM radios included. If you put "pedometer" or "10,000 steps" into a search engine like Google, you will get lots of options and information.

How can I exercise safely without developing a low blood glucose (hypoglycemia)?

The most important things to do to keep safe are to tune in to how your body feels and check your blood glucose frequently. Always check your blood glucose before you start to exercise. If your blood glucose is under 100 mg/dL (5.6 mmol/L), you should eat some carbohydrate before you start your exercise. If you are exercising for more than half an hour, you should stop and check your blood glucose during your exercise. Checking soon after you finish and then again an hour or so later will help you to get a sense of how your blood glucose changes during particular types and amounts of exercise. You should have glucose (tablets, juice, regular pop, or "sports drinks") available while you exercise, as well as more long-lasting carbohydrate snacks, especially if you plan to do prolonged exercise.

Why does exercise have a bigger effect on my blood glucose in the afternoon than it does in the morning?

Most of us are more resistant to insulin in the early morning than we are later in the day. In the hours before we wake up, our bodies prepare for the day by pushing hormones like cortisol and growth hormone into our blood. These hormones make it harder for insulin to help glucose to get out of our blood and into our muscles. You can test your blood glucose before, during, and after the same amount of exercise at the same time every day or at different times of the day. You will probably find that when you exercise at the same time every day, you get more predictable changes in your blood glucose. For most people, doing the same amount of exercise in the afternoon or evening causes the blood glucose to drop more than doing the same amount of exercise in the morning. It also depends on when you last ate and when you took your diabetes pills or insulin.

Why does my blood glucose sometimes drop several hours after I have finished exercising?

We all store in our muscle cells an extra supply of "glucose energy" in the form of a substance called glycogen. When you exercise vigorously, you use up the store of glycogen in your muscles in about half an hour. If you keep exercising, then your muscles will send out signals to say, "Feed me!" Your blood glucose might drop, and you might feel hypoglycemic. You might eat snacks of carbohydrate to keep your blood glucose up. In addition, your liver releases glucose from its store of glycogen, and so your muscles are kept supplied with energy while you exercise. When you finish exercising, your blood glucose might be fine (well over 100 mg/dL, or 5.6 mmol/L). You might even have a meal or a snack to keep your blood glucose up. But for the next six to ten hours, your muscles will continue to suck glucose out of your blood to replenish their stores of muscle glycogen. This is especially noticeable after really prolonged exercise (like running a marathon or doing several hours of cycling or basketball). This can cause episodes of severe hypoglycemia several hours after you stop your exercise.

Why does my blood glucose sometimes go up instead of down after exercise?

This can be really confusing. You expect that when you exercise, your muscles will use up glucose, and so your blood glucose level should drop. The effect of exercise on your blood glucose depends on how much insulin you have in your system at the time of your exercise. If you have plenty of insulin in your blood along with the glucose, then your blood glucose will drop with exercise. However, if you are someone who takes insulin and your last insulin shot is wearing off, you might get a surprise.

I see this most often in people who take two shots a day of a medium-acting insulin like NPH. They took a shot the previous evening and want to exercise first thing in the morning, before they have taken their morning shot. If the insulin from the previous evening's shot has worn off, their blood glucose might already be high and rising. Now, when they exercise, their muscles use up their supply of muscle glycogen and then send signals that they need more glucose. Glucose gets released from the liver, and so the blood glucose rises. But if there is too little insulin around, then the glucose cannot get out of the blood and into the muscles. When that happens, you will probably feel exhausted during your workout and will be surprised to find that your blood glucose at the end is higher than it was to start with.

If you check your blood glucose before you start to exercise and it is over 250 mg/dL (13.9 mmol/L), then you should probably take your insulin or pills and wait until your blood glucose is down below 200 mg/dL (11.1 mmol/L) before you start to exercise.

Chapter 19

Stress and Diabetes

- What causes stress?
- Why does stress affect my blood glucose so much?
- Why does stress sometimes make my blood glucose go down instead of up?
- What can I do to reduce my stress?
- Does a fever raise your blood glucose?
- Do stress and diabetes give you a higher chance of getting a yeast infection?
- Are blood glucose levels affected by your menstrual cycle?
- Can chemotherapy drugs affect diabetes?

What causes stress?

Anytime your body is not "happy" about something, it gets stressed. If you are in pain, if you injure yourself or break a bone, your body gets stressed. If you get an infection in your throat, ear, bladder, skin, lungs, or anywhere in your body, it causes stress. If you are too cold or too hot or wet or starving, your body gets stressed. And if you are angry or unhappy or worried or scared, that can be stressful to your body, too. So everything from physical injury to psychological problems can cause stress.

Funnily enough, your body responds to all of these different kinds of stress in a very similar way. It releases large amounts of the hormones adrenaline (also called epinephrine), noradrenaline (or norepinephrine), glucagon, cortisol, and growth hormone. These are sometimes called the "stress hormones." They act in different ways to raise the glucose level in your blood by encouraging glucose to be released from your liver. They make it harder for insulin to work properly, and so they make your body more resistant to the effects of insulin.

Why does stress affect my blood glucose so much?

Stress can have an enormous effect on your blood glucose. Whatever the cause of the stress, your body responds by pushing a variety of hormones like adrenaline, cortisol, growth hormone, and glucagon out into your bloodstream. All of these hormones counteract the effects of insulin and so make your body more resistant to insulin. This means that your body needs to put out more insulin to overcome the resistance. If your body is not able to do this because you have diabetes, then your blood glucose will rise. The other reason why stress can cause a rise in blood glucose is because when we are stressed, we tend to eat more and exercise less. If the stress in your life never seems to let up, you may need to ask your doctor for some help. You may benefit from counseling or some medication to lower your stress and anxiety. You may need an increase in your diabetes pills, or you may need to take some insulin shots in addition to the pills, depending on how high the blood glucose is and how it responds to the other things that you try.

Why does stress sometimes make my blood glucose go down instead of up?

Although this is less common than blood glucose going up with stress, it can sometimes go down. If you are stressed about an upcoming exam or test or job interview, you may release a lot of adrenaline and feel very "hyper" and agitated. Some people can't sit still when they are stressed. They forget to eat. They rush around cleaning up and tidying and doing tasks to take their mind off the stressful situation. If that is how you respond to stress, then it is quite possible that your blood glucose will go down instead of up.

What can I do to reduce my stress?

Obviously, there is no easy answer to this. Entire books are written on the topic. Many people make their living counseling others on stress-reduction techniques. The first thing to do is to understand what is causing your stress. If it is painful joints from arthritis or an infection in your lungs, then you need to get treatment to reduce the pain or heal the infection. If it is a specific psychological problem such as an unpleasant work environment or a bad relationship, then you need to consider options such as changing jobs or getting out of the bad relationship. If your whole life just seems too busy and too stressful, then it can be harder to identify any specific one or two things for you to change. Talk it over with your friends. Try to find some time every day to do something nice for yourself. If you find that you respond to stress by doing unhealthy things like overeating on "comfort " food or drinking too much alcohol, then you should get professional help from a behavioral health therapist or a psychological counselor.

Does a fever raise your blood glucose?

Yes, it can. A fever is a sign that your body is under stress, fighting off an infection or some other illness. Just like with other forms of stress, your body will respond by pushing out lots of "stress hormones" that make it harder for insulin to work properly, and so your blood glucose will go up.

Do stress and diabetes give you a higher chance of getting a yeast infection?

Yes, they do. People without diabetes are more likely to get yeast infections when they are stressed. If you have diabetes, you are even more likely to get yeast infections, especially if your average blood glucose levels are high or you are stressed or both.

Are blood glucose levels affected by your menstrual cycle?

Yes, they are. In the week before your menstrual period starts, you have high levels of hormones like progesterone in your blood. You may also feel bloated and swollen with extra fluid that week and might feel some pain or discomfort in your abdomen. All of these things cause stress to your body and make it harder for insulin to work properly. If you find that your blood glucose levels are a lot higher in the week before your period, you should talk to your doctor about making changes to your diabetes treatment that week. I know quite a few young women with diabetes who need to increase their doses of insulin during the week before their period starts and then have to cut back the doses again as soon as their period starts.

Can chemotherapy drugs affect diabetes?

Very much so. Usually getting chemotherapy to treat cancer puts a big stress on your body, and so your blood glucose levels might go up a lot. But sometimes the chemotherapy drugs make you feel so nauseated that you hardly feel like eating at all, and so you may need less insulin or other diabetes treatment when you are getting chemotherapy. It depends on what particular chemotherapy drugs you are getting and how bad you feel while you are getting them. The best advice I can give you for a situation like this is to make sure you drink plenty of fluids while you are getting chemotherapy and check your blood glucose frequently.

Chapter 20

Drugs for Type 2 Diabetes

- Can diabetes be fixed with pills?
- Will my new diabetes medicine cause me to gain weight?
- How do I know which drugs are best when there are so many choices?
- Why does my doctor not use the same diabetes medicine on me that my neighbor's doctor prescribes for her?

Can diabetes be fixed with pills?

It depends on what type of diabetes you have and what else you are doing to help yourself stay healthy. If you have type 1 diabetes, your body will make no insulin at all, and so you will need to take insulin by injection. Insulin does not come as a pill. If you have type 2 diabetes, there are many different types of pill that can help you. Some of them make your pancreas push out more insulin; others make you more responsive (or less resistant) to insulin. Some of them slow down the way your body absorbs carbohydrate or fat from your guts. But none of the pills or injectable drugs will "fix" your diabetes completely. They won't work very well if you don't make any changes to what you eat and how you exercise. But there are some very effective pills that will help you keep your diabetes well controlled if you are also making healthy changes to your lifestyle.

Will my new diabetes medicine cause me to gain weight?

It depends. There are two main reasons why you might gain weight. If your body holds onto more water than it should, you will retain fluid, and that can cause weight gain. When this happens, you may notice some ankle swelling. If it is severe, you may notice you are thicker around your middle and might even get breathless. You should check with your doctor if you think you are swelling up with fluid. Certain diabetes pills (like rosiglitazone [Avandia] and pioglitazone [Actos]) can cause your body to hold onto a lot of fluid. Although fluid retention could be caused by one of your diabetes pills, there are other problems that can cause you to retain fluid, so you should talk to your doctor about it.

The other way to gain weight is when your body makes more fat. None of the diabetic medicines, including insulin, will *make* you gain weight. The only way you gain weight is if you are eating more calories than you are using up in your daily life and activities. But some diabetes medicines make it harder than others to keep your weight off. If a diabetes medicine makes your pancreas push insulin into your blood all day long, even between meals, then your blood glucose may drop, and you may feel hungry and need to eat. Also, if your blood glucose has been high for a while, your kidneys will filter glucose out of your blood and into your urine. You may be losing several hundred calories a day down the toilet. If you start a new diabetes medicine that brings your blood glucose down, you will stop losing those extra calories in your urine. If you don't start eating less, you will begin to gain weight.

How do I know which drugs are best when there are so many choices?

It is difficult to know what drugs are best for you without knowing more details about your diabetes. There are many good options. Your doctor should be able to help you. Some drugs are much more expensive than others, but this does not mean that they are always better. Drug companies do a lot of advertising directly to consumers on television, in magazines, or on the internet. You will be bombarded with ads for new diabetes drugs. They always sound as if they are much better than the older drugs, but that is not always true.

Sometimes it takes years before all of the side effects and problems associated with a new drug get discovered. It may be a good idea to stick to drugs that have been around for a long time. It depends on your personality. Some people like to take risks and always prefer the newest thing. Other people are more cautious.

Why does my doctor not use the same diabetes medicines on me that my neighbor's doctor prescribes for her?

One possibility is that you and your neighbor have different types of diabetes or are at different stages of your diabetes or have different other medical conditions. You may need different combinations of drugs. Another possibility is that your doctor and your neighbor's doctor have different opinions about which drugs they think are best. Doctors all have different personalities, too. Some doctors like to prescribe the newest drugs, while others are more cautious.

You should ask a lot of questions about any drug that you are being prescribed or are thinking about taking. How does it work? How long has it been on the market? How expensive is it? What are the side effects? You need to make an educated decision. If a drug is likely to do a lot more good than harm to you, then it is worth taking. If you don't have enough information to make that decision, then you might want to hold off until you know more.

Chapter 21

Insulin Resistance Drugs

- How does metformin work?
- What are the benefits of using metformin?
- What are the problems with metformin?
- Why use an old-fashioned drug like metformin when there are more modern options?
- How do the glitazones work?
- What are the benefits of using a glitazone?
- What are the problems with the glitazones?

How does metformin work?

Metformin (U.S. brand names Glucophage, Glucophage XR, Fortamet, Glumetza, Riomet) has been used for over forty years around the world, so we know a lot about it. It only works if your body makes some insulin. One of the reasons why the blood glucose stays so high when you have type 2 diabetes is because your liver releases too much glucose from its stores into your blood. Metformin makes your liver respond better to insulin so that you push less glucose out of your liver into your blood. Metformin also helps your muscles and other organs to respond to insulin better, and so they take more glucose out of your blood to use as energy.

What are the benefits of using metformin?

Metformin does not raise the amount of insulin in your body. People tend to feel less hungry, rather than more hungry, when they take it, and so their weight is likely to stay the same, even though their blood glucose comes down. On average it will help drop your blood glucose by about 20 percent when you start using it. So if your blood glucose average was 200 mg/dL (11.1 mmol/L) before you start metformin, it is likely to be about 160 mg/dL (8.9 mmol/L) after a few months on metformin. Metformin can be used along with other pills or insulin. These combinations usually result in even bigger improvements in blood glucose.

What are the problems with metformin?

Metformin pills are large (either 500 mg or 850 mg size). Most people need to take three or four pills a day (up to 2,500 mg) to get the full effect of the drug. It can cause an upset stomach in some people (an ache in the abdomen, nausea, a metallic taste in the mouth, or diarrhea). This is more likely if the dose is started too high and if it is taken on an empty stomach. It is best to start at a low dose (maybe even half of a 500 mg pill taken with food) for a few days and build the dose up slowly.

Metformin does not damage the heart or liver or kidneys, but they all need to be working well in order for you to be able to clear metformin out of your system. You should have a blood test called serum creatinine done once or twice a year while you are taking metformin. This test tells us how well your kidneys are working. Your doctor may also do a blood test to check how well your liver is working and may also examine your heart. If metformin is not cleared out of your body well enough, then lactic acid can build up inside your body, causing a rare but serious condition called lactic acidosis.

Why use an old-fashioned drug like metformin when there are more modern options?

Metformin is the only member of a class of drug called biguanides. Drug companies have tried to develop other drugs in this class, but none have been found to be as effective or safe as metformin. It is available in generic forms and so is relatively cheap. It works well along with many other classes of drug. So despite the fact that there are many newer drugs available, most doctors agree that metformin is a good drug to start with if you have type 2 diabetes and you can't keep your blood glucose where you want it with changes to your eating and exercise alone. Adding metformin will usually bring your HbA1c down by at least one whole percentage point without causing any weight gain.

One of the biggest problems with a lot of the newer drugs is that we don't have long term studies telling us if the new drug will actually do you good if you take it for years on end. New drugs are often heavily advertised. The pharmaceutical companies often gloss over potential problems and stress only the possible benefits of taking their drug. We often don't hear about side effects until many years after a drug is on the market.

The story of troglitazone (Rezulin) is one that everyone ought to think about before they take a new drug too enthusiastically. Rezulin was a new "wonder drug" for type 2 diabetes that hit the U.S. market in January 1997. Hundreds of my patients who were taking metformin asked if they could be switched to Rezulin. It was a smaller pill, easier to take, and didn't cause the stomachache and loose bowels that some people get with metformin. The problem was that there was a lot of concern in the early research studies that Rezulin caused severe liver damage in some patients and that this could continue even after stopping the drug. The drug company who made Rezulin kept fighting to keep it on the market, and so it remained on the market until March 2000, despite the fact that more and more people were dying from liver failure.

Don't get me wrong. There are some incredibly beneficial breakthrough drugs that come on the market every few years, but truthfully, there aren't as many as you might think. A good example of a new class of drugs that has dramatically improved the health of many people is the statin drugs for lowering cholesterol and reducing the risk of heart attacks and strokes. When the first of those drugs (lovastatin, or Mevacor) hit the markets about twenty years ago, some doctors were very skeptical about it. But now that tens of thousands of people have been studied in randomized, controlled trials and have been followed for five to ten years using outcomes that really matter to people like you and me (outcomes like "are you more or less likely to die or have a heart attack taking this drug?"), it is clear that the statin drugs truly cause more good than harm.

How do the glitazones work?

The glitazones are also called thiazolidinediones, or TZDs. The original TZD was called troglitazone (Rezulin) but has been taken off the market because it caused serious liver damage. There are two glitazones still on the market called rosiglitazone (Avandia) and pioglitazone (Actos). They work by going right inside cells that respond to insulin (like fat cells and muscle cells), where they make those cells respond to insulin better. They make it easier for glucose to be taken inside fat cells and muscle cells, where it can be used. It often takes several weeks before the full effect of a glitazone is seen on the blood glucose. The glitazones do many other things in the body. They change some of the lipid (fat) levels in the blood. They make it harder for your body to make new bone tissue.

What are the benefits of using a glitazone?

They are easy to take as a small pill, once or twice a day. They do not cause stomach upset or diarrhea, which can be a problem with some of the other drugs that I have mentioned. They can work along with other pills and insulin to reduce blood glucose. If your blood glucose is still too high, even though you are trying to do the best you can with diet and exercise and taking other pills, and if you really want to put off using insulin for as long as possible, then adding a glitazone might help. When glitazones have been given to people with impaired glucose tolerance, they delayed the onset of type 2 diabetes by a couple of years. It is not clear whether they can actually prevent anyone from ever getting type 2 diabetes or whether they just delay it.

What are the problems with the glitazones?

In the ten years since these drugs came on the market, the number of problems and side effects that we know about has grown. Troglitazone (Rezulin) was taken off the market, because it caused very serious liver damage that has resulted in several deaths. Because of this, if you are taking rosiglitazone (Avandia) or pioglitazone (Actos), you will be asked to get a blood test from time to time to check your liver. They can cause your body to retain fluid. This can cause ankle swelling and can sometimes be enough to cause heart failure. Heart failure occurs when the heart is not able to pump hard enough, and so fluid can "dam back" in the lungs, causing breathlessness, or in the abdomen or legs, causing weight gain or ankle swelling. Heart failure can be very serious.

The glitazones also cause weight gain because they encourage your body to make new fat cells. You have fat cells throughout your body, including inside your abdomen and under your skin. The glitazones cause you to put more of the fat under your skin. They also prevent your body from making new bone cells. This can cause bone thinning (osteoporosis) that can make some people more likely to fracture their bones.

Chapter 22

Insulin Production Drugs

- How do sulfonylureas work?
- What are the benefits of using sulfonylureas?
- What are the problems with sulfonylureas?
- What are the advantages of the newer meglitinides?

How do sulfonylureas work?

Sulfonylureas are another old-fashioned drug. They were originally developed in the 1950s as antibiotics, but when it was discovered that they caused hypoglycemia (low blood glucose), they became used to treat diabetes. They act on receptors on the islet cells in the pancreas to force those cells to push out more insulin. The first sulfonylureas to be made, like chlorpropamide (U.S. brand name Diabinese) and tolbutamide (Tolinase), were larger pills (250 or 500 mg). They are sometimes called "first generation sulfonylureas."

The newer sulfonylureas, which are sometimes called second or third generation drugs, are more powerful and so come in smaller pills (1, 2, 5, or 10 mg). These include glyburide (DiaBeta, Micronase, Glynase, Pres Tab) or glipizide (Glucotrol, Glucotrol XL) or glimepiride (Amaryl). They mostly vary from each other in how big a dose you need, how long they hang around in your body after you take a pill, and how expensive they are. Most of them are generic, and so they are fairly inexpensive. Because they force your pancreas to push out insulin, they help to bring your blood glucose down.

What are the benefits of using sulfonylureas?

The sulfonylureas are inexpensive and work quickly. You will see the effects the first day that you use them. Some other drugs, like metformin and the glitazones, take several days or weeks before the full effect is seen. Sulfonylureas work well along with other drugs and insulin to bring the blood glucose down.

What are the problems with sulfonylureas?

Because they were derived from sulfonamide drugs, they can cause a variety of skin reactions in people who have a sulfa-allergy. They can cause an itchy, red skin rash that gets worse when you are exposed to the sun. Hypoglycemia (low blood glucose) can also be a problem, especially with very long-lasting sulfonylureas like chlorpropamide and glyburide. You need to carry glucose and other carbohydrates with you and be ready to use them if you feel symptoms of low blood glucose (sweating, shakiness, hunger, anxiety). Because of this, you may gain weight after taking sulfonylureas for several months, especially if they are causing you to feel hungry and shaky between meals. Some of the sulfonylureas can cause fluid retention. There is a long list of other possible side effects, but these are less common.

What are the advantages of the newer meglitinides?

Both repaglinide (Prandin) and nateglinide (Starlix) are newer drugs that also stimulate the islet cells in your pancreas to push out more insulin. They are more expensive than the sulfonylureas but have two advantages. Since they are not derived from sulfa-drugs, they can be taken even if you have a sulfa-allergy or get skin rashes with a sulfonylurea. They are shorter-acting and do not cause your islets to push out so much insulin between meals. Because of this, they are a bit less likely to cause hypoglycemia in between meals.

Chapter 23 OTHER DRUGS

- How does acarbose work?
- What are the benefits of using acarbose?
- What are the problems with acarbose?
- How does orlistat work?
- What are the benefits of using orlistat?
- What are the problems with orlistat?
- How does exenatide (Byetta) work?
- What are the benefits of using exenatide (Byetta)?
- What are the problems with exenatide (Byetta)?
- How does sitagliptin (Januvia) work?
- What are the benefits of using sitagliptin (Januvia)?
- What are the problems with sitagliptin (Januvia)?
- What other drugs are in development for type 2 diabetes?

How does acarbose work?

Acarbose (Precose) is a drug that you take as a pill with the first bite of your main meals. It mixes with your food so that when your food leaves your stomach, the acarbose slows down the digestion of complex carbohydrates like bread and starches. Normally, your pancreas and guts secrete enzymes (like amylase, maltase, and isomaltase), which very quickly break down complex carbohydrates into smaller molecules like glucose, which then get absorbed into your blood. This is why your blood glucose rises within minutes of eating bread or potatoes. Acarbose stops these enzymes from working so fast, and so it takes much longer for the carbohydrate to be digested and absorbed. Another drug called miglitol (Glyset) works in a similar way to acarbose. Because acarbose slows down carbohydrate digestion, your blood glucose rises much slower after a meal. This gives the insulin in your body more time to deal with the glucose, and so your blood glucose does not swing so high immediately after a meal or swing so low a few hours later.

What are the benefits of using acarbose?

Because acarbose works inside your gut and is not absorbed into your body, it is a safe drug with very few serious side effects. It does not cause weight gain. It has been used to treat people with impaired glucose tolerance and has been shown to delay the onset of diabetes by a few years. Acarbose can also be used along with other pills and with insulin to treat diabetes.

What are the problems with acarbose?

Because acarbose delays the absorption of complex carbohydrate, some of that carbohydrate can travel all the way down your small intestines and arrive in your colon (your large bowel) without being absorbed. The bacteria in your colon can then ferment that carbohydrate and this can cause you to make a lot of wind and diarrhea.

Using acarbose is a bit like eating a diet that contains a lot of beans, lentils, and onions. For some people, the embarrassment of passing smelly gas that other people may notice makes it too unpleasant to take. These side effects are worse at higher doses of acarbose (100 mg or 200 mg per day) and are much less noticeable at doses of 25 or 50 mg per day. Unfortunately, at these lower doses, acarbose only has a small effect on lowering your blood glucose. Acarbose can cause hypoglycemia. Because it prevents your body from breaking down complex carbohydrate, you must be sure to take glucose and not juice, table sugar, bread, or crackers to treat your hypoglycemic symptoms.

How does orlistat work?

Orlistat (Xenical) is another drug that blocks some of the enzymes in your guts. Orlistat inhibits the enzyme lipase, which helps your body to break down fat into smaller pieces that get absorbed into your body. Because it stops you from digesting and absorbing so much fat in your diet, it can help you to lose weight. Every gram of fat that you eat gives you 9 calories, but when you are taking orlistat, a lot of that fat stays in your bowels and gets flushed down the toilet.

What are the benefits of using orlistat?

Orlistat can help you to lose weight and lower your blood glucose. It can be used along with other pills and insulin in combination.

What are the problems with orlistat?

Because it prevents you from absorbing fat, you tend to have diarrhea with unpleasant smelly, fatty bowel movements. It can prevent you from absorbing certain vitamins and can sometimes cause an inflammation of the pancreas. The effects on weight loss also tend to go away over time. Most people have lost most of the weight they will lose by six months, and even after continuing to use orlistat for one or two years, many people regain part or all of the weight. One reason for this is that people figure out that if they eat less fat in their diet and replace it with more carbohydrate, then their bowel movements become less unpleasant and less frequent. But by eating more carbohydrate instead of fat, they absorb more calories and so regain their weight.

How does exenatide (Byetta) work?

In the lower part of our intestines, we make a hormone called "glucagon-like polypeptide number 1" (GLP-1). This helps your pancreas to push out insulin. It slows down how fast our stomach empties after a meal. It makes us feel satisfied after a meal and helps insulin to work better. If you have type 2 diabetes, you make less GLP-1 than you should. This is one of the reasons why your blood glucose rises so much after meals. GLP-1 does not stay around very long in your blood. You break it down using an enzyme called *dipeptidyl peptidase number 4* (DPP-IV).

Exenatide (Byetta) is a naturally occurring compound that is found in the saliva of the Gila monster, a venomous lizard (so exenatide is sometimes referred to as the "lizard spit" drug!). Exenatide works like a long-lasting form of GLP-1, because it is not destroyed by DPP-IV. It has to be given by an injection under the skin twice a day. It works to help you release insulin from your own pancreas. It also slows your stomach emptying and makes you feel more satisfied after a meal.

What are the benefits of using exenatide (Byetta)?

Like so many new drugs on the market, we don't know the true answer to this. We do not know whether using exenatide for many years will cause more good than harm. It often takes five or ten years until many thousands of people have used it before we know the answer to that. What we do know is that when you start taking exenatide, you may notice that you are less hungry, and so it is easier to eat the right amount of food. You may find that your blood glucose does not rise so fast after a meal and that your blood glucose comes down faster. You may need to reduce your dose of other diabetes pills or insulin when you start taking exenatide. Some people lose weight after starting exenatide, although we don't have much information yet about how long this lasts and how many patients are able to keep their weight off several years later.

What are the problems with exenatide (Byetta)?

Many people feel a little nauseated when they start taking exenatide. It is recommended to start at 5 mcg twice a day for the first few weeks and only increase to 10 mcg twice a day once you are used to it. Some people find that it makes them feel so sick that they vomit. Hypoglycemia (low blood glucose) is another major problem for some people, although that can usually be managed by reducing the dose of other diabetic pills or insulin. Exenatide can also cause a severe inflammation of the pancreas (pancreatitis) in some people. This is a very serious complication that can cause severe pain in your abdomen requiring emergency treatment in the hospital. We will not yet know if there are more long term problems with exenatide until more people have been on it for longer.

How does sitagliptin (Januvia) work?

Sitagliptin is a drug that prevents the DPP-IV from breaking down the GLP-1 that your own body makes. It is the first drug in a new class of drugs called DPP-IV inhibitors. It can be taken as a pill, so you do not need to take injections under the skin to get the effect of sitagliptin. It helps the level of GLP-1 in your own blood to stay higher and for longer than usual. This should help you to push out more insulin, use it more effectively, and slow down your stomach emptying.

What are the benefits of using sitagliptin (Januvia)?

Like so many new drugs on the market, we don't know the true answer to this. We do not know whether using sitagliptin for many years will cause more good than harm. It often takes five or ten years until many thousands of people have used it before we know the answer to that. Sitagliptin is an easy drug to take, because it is a pill that you take once a day. The effects of sitagliptin are not nearly as dramatic as they are with exenatide. You are not likely to lose weight, and the improvement in blood glucose is more modest. However, if added to other treatment, it will help your blood glucose to get lower.

What are the problems with sitagliptin (Januvia)?

We do not know all of the side effects. Like many drugs, it can cause allergic skin reactions in some people. It can also cause nausea and stomach ache. Some people get a headache with it. A more worrying symptom is that using sitagliptin may increase your risk of nose, throat, and sinus infections. We do not know whether more side effects and problems will be discovered when many thousands of people are put on it and followed for years.

What other drugs are in development for type 2 diabetes?

There are many new drugs in development. Several companies are working on other DPP-IV inhibitors. There may be other thiazolidinediones. There are several new approaches being tried to help with weight loss.

Chapter 24

Going on Insulin

- My doctor says I need insulin now. Is this my fault?
- My doctor says I need insulin. Does that mean my diabetes is getting worse?
- I knew someone who went on insulin and died a month later, so does that mean insulin must be bad for you?
- When is insulin a good idea for someone with type 2 diabetes?
- Once you go on insulin, can you ever come off it again?
- Why can't insulin be given as a pill?
- Won't insulin make me gain weight?

My doctor says I need insulin now. Is this my fault?

Absolutely not. I get so sad when people think that if they need to go onto insulin that they have somehow "failed" and that if they had done something differently, they wouldn't need insulin. Yes, it is possible that if you ate even less and exercised more that you could possibly put off the time when you need to start taking insulin, but I see people putting off the use of insulin much too long. It usually gets harder to keep your glucose level in a good range when you have type 2 diabetes. Over time your body simply makes less and less insulin. There is not much that you can do to stop that process. It is "in your genes," and that is not your fault.

My doctor says I need insulin. Does that mean my diabetes is getting worse?

Not really. If your body is making less insulin, then giving yourself insulin to replace what you don't make is a very sensible approach. The thing that causes damage to your body is how high your blood glucose stays over years. Yes, it may be harder to keep your blood glucose in range right now, and so adding insulin may make it seem as though your diabetes is getting worse; but if you add insulin and keep your blood glucose in a good range, then you will be less likely to have problems from your diabetes, not more likely.

I knew someone who went on insulin and died a month later, so does that mean insulin must be bad for you?

Not at all. A lot of people have some kind of horror story like this from a friend or neighbor. It is not likely that starting insulin caused the person's death. It may be that by the time the insulin was started, the person was very ill. Think of taking insulin as taking the natural hormone supplement that your body doesn't make quite enough of. Compared to many of the drugs that are used to treat diabetes, insulin has very few side effects, indeed. It is a very natural way to treat a condition where the problem is that you don't make enough insulin.

When is insulin a good idea for someone with type 2 diabetes?

If you are doing the best you can to eat healthy and to get exercise, but you find that your blood glucose first thing in the morning (your fasting blood glucose) is too high no matter what you do, then adding some insulin at bedtime can be very helpful. I usually advise my patients to work on their lifestyle first, and if that is not enough, then I add metformin and build that up until their fasting blood glucose average is below 120 mg/dL (6.7 mmol/L) and their HbA1c is under 7.0 percent. If lifestyle and metformin are not enough to do this, then I will discuss with them whether to add another pill or whether to add a shot of long-acting insulin at that point.

Many people choose to add insulin and get great results. Compared with adding a sulfonylurea, a meglitinides, or a glitazone to the metformin, when you add bedtime insulin and adjust the dose to get the fasting blood glucose average below 120 mg/dL (6.7 mmol/L), you get less weight gain, less hypoglycemia, and a lower HbA1c. It is a very good approach for a lot of people.

Once you go on insulin, can you ever come off it again?

Yes, you can, although very few people want to. I have met hundreds of people over the years who have put off starting insulin for years because of fears that if they ever went onto insulin, they were admitting defeat, and they could never come off it again. When they finally let me persuade them to try adding some insulin, the most common response I hear a few months later is, "Wow, I feel so much better! I wish I had done it years ago." For anyone who does not feel like that, I simply stop the insulin again. Their blood glucose levels and their symptoms just go back to the way they were before the insulin was started.

Why can't insulin be given as a pill?

Insulin is a protein molecule. If you take it by mouth, your stomach acid and the digestive enzymes in your guts will very quickly chop it up into bits that you absorb into your body, just like you would a piece of meat that you eat. So the insulin doesn't get a chance to have any effect on your blood glucose at all. Scientists and doctors have tried wrapping insulin in a protective coating to stop it from being chewed up by the acid and enzymes in your guts, but that approach has not been successful. You could give insulin as a skin patch, but it causes too much skin irritation. Insulin is absorbed when you inhale it into your lungs, but as I will discuss later, there are problems with inhaled insulin, too.

Won't insulin make me gain weight?

Not necessarily. The only way anyone gains weight (apart from retaining fluid, that is) is by taking more calories into your body (over days, weeks, and months) than you are burning up with activity and exercise. If you take too big of a dose of insulin or take the wrong type of insulin, it may make you hypoglycemic and hungry so that you eat more than your body needs. In that case, you will gain weight. But if you only take the right amount of the right kind of insulin, and if you continue to eat the right amount of food and get enough exercise, then you will not gain weight with insulin.

Chapter 25 INSULIN BASICS

- Do people with type 1 diabetes always need insulin?
- How do they make insulin?
- Why are some types of insulin cloudy?
- How many types of insulin are there?
- Why should I take more than one type of insulin?
- How high a dose of insulin can you give?
- How can I decide what the best types of insulin are for me?
- What are the differences between the fast-acting insulins?
- How soon before a meal should I inject my fast-acting insulin?
- How do you decide how much fast-acting insulin to give before a meal?
- Isn't if better to give the insulin after the meal, when you know how high the blood glucose has gone?
- Is it ever okay to inject insulin after the meal?
- What are the differences between the longer-acting insulins?
- How do you choose the right size of insulin syringe and needle?
- Should my spouse or close friend know how to give me my shot?
- How often should I change the needle on my syringe or pen?
- Should I swab my skin with alcohol before injecting myself?
- Where is the best place on my body to inject insulin?
- What is the best system for rotating my insulin shots?

Do people with type 1 diabetes always need insulin?

Yes. When you are first diagnosed with type 1 diabetes, your own pancreas is still able to make some insulin. But the islet cells in the pancreas are under attack by your own immune system. By the time you are diagnosed, you may already have destroyed three-quarters of your insulin-producing islet cells. The ones that remain are not working very well. The high level of glucose in your blood drives your islet cells to push out as much insulin as they can, but all the time, they are being attacked by poisons made by the immune cells (lymphocytes) nearby.

Once you start taking insulin shots and your blood glucose comes down, this takes pressure off your struggling islet cells, so they recover for a while and are able to push out more insulin. Sometimes they recover so well that you can be taken off insulin again for several weeks or even for a few months. Doctors used to do this routinely. After you had just gotten used to the idea of having diabetes and taking insulin for the rest of your life, your diabetes appeared to go away and your insulin was stopped.

Instead of stopping insulin in the first few months, it is much smarter to keep taking insulin to get your blood glucose levels as close to normal as you can. By doing this, you are protecting yourself from getting damage to your body from a high blood glucose. You are also slowing down the rate at which the rest of your islet cells get destroyed. If you keep your diabetes well controlled from the start, you can continue making some insulin of your own for several years. You might think, "So what? Why should I care? I am taking insulin shots anyway." But if your body can still make a little insulin of its own, it means that your blood glucose levels are easier to control and don't swing about so unpredictably.

How do they make insulin?

Until the 1980s, the only way to get insulin was to grind up the pancreas of thousands of cows and pigs in slaughterhouses and extract the insulin from them. Insulin is a molecule made up of fifty-one smaller building blocks called amino acids. As I showed in Figure 1 on page 6, these are arranged in two chains. The A-chain contains twenty-one amino acids, and the B-chain contains thirty. Insulin from cattle is almost identical to human insulin. Forty-eight of those amino acids are exactly the same and in the same place as human insulin. Only three amino acids are different. With pig insulin, only one amino acid is different from human insulin.

Insulin from animals worked very well, especially when techniques improved for cleaning out traces of other material that could contaminate the insulin that got put into bottles. But even highly purified animal insulin could still be recognized by your body as "foreign." As a result, allergy to insulin could sometimes cause skin rashes, ugly hollowed out sections in the fat under your skin (a condition called lipoatrophy), and high antibody levels that could slow down the effects of insulin. It was thought that human insulin would be better. One way to make human insulin was to take pig insulin and remove the amino acid at the end of the B-chain and replace it with the amino acid that humans have in that position. For several years this was done. But with advances in molecular biology, it became possible to identify the exact structure of DNA for the gene that makes human insulin. Scientists then inserted the human insulin gene into bacteria. When those bacteria doubled and doubled and grew into millions and billions, they became little human insulin–making factories.

Now almost all of the insulin that is used around the world is made in massive vats of bacteria. This means that we can make as much as we need, and because it is identical to the insulin that our own bodies make, it causes less of an allergic reaction. It is interesting that we can still become allergic to human insulin, though. This may be due to traces of other chemicals and preservatives in the bottles or because our bodies are not used to having insulin being injected into the fat under our skin. But for most people, injecting human insulin under the skin works extremely well.

Why are some types of insulin cloudy?

Adding protamine (a fish protein) or zinc to insulin makes it cloudy. In the middle of the twentieth century, scientists found that if they added these substances to the mixture, they could slow down how quickly insulin was absorbed from your subcutaneous fat into your blood. So they made insulin zinc suspensions. At the Hagedorn laboratory in Gentofte, just outside Copenhagen in Denmark, they added protamine to insulin. This mixture was quite acidic, and so they adjusted the mixture until it was at a neutral pH. The insulin was called Neutral Protamine insulin from the Hagedorn laboratories, or NPH insulin. This is still one of the most popular insulins on the market today.

Insulin that has nothing else added to it and has not been modified in any way is sometimes called Regular insulin. When you inject Regular insulin under your skin, it begins to be absorbed into your blood in twenty to thirty minutes. The amount of insulin in your blood continues to rise over the next two to four hours and then declines over the next two to four hours. In other words, Regular insulin has its onset in twenty to thirty minutes, its peak in two to four hours, and a duration of six to eight hours. So if Regular insulin was the only type of insulin available, you would need to give yourself four shots a day—one shot every six hours. The insulin level would rise and fall four times; you would need to eat in the middle of each of the four peaks, or your blood glucose would drop too low.

Imagine doing that and not even being able to check your blood glucose, so you never knew what it was until you felt yourself getting too low.

Many people still refer to their insulins as "clear" (fast-acting) and "cloudy" (longer). Another shorthand that some people use is to call the fast-acting insulin "R" (since most brands of Regular insulin have a large R on the bottle) and the longer-acting insulin "N." Nowadays, those shorthand terms are becoming more and more misleading, I'm afraid, because there are many new clear preparations of insulin that are much faster acting than Regular insulin and a couple that are much slower acting than the cloudy insulins.

How many types of insulin are there?

There are more and more every year. Several different pharmaceutical companies make human Regular insulin and NPH insulin. Sometimes they combine different amounts of R and N in the same bottle (so there is a "70/30" insulin that contains 70 percent of NPH mixed with 30 percent of Regular, for example). There are also a growing number of insulin analogs on the market. Scientists have tinkered with the human insulin molecule in ways that either speed up or slow down the rate at which it is absorbed from under your skin into your blood. The table on the next page shows some of the most common insulins on the market, along with a rough idea of when they start to work (their onset), when they have their peak, and how long they last (their duration). You will see that I have put quite a big range in for each of these. There is a lot of variation in how fast different people absorb the same amount of the same kind of insulin. There is also a lot of variation in how the same person absorbs the same amount of the same kind of insulin from one day to the next. I will explain more about that later and why it matters.

Insulin type	Onset	Peak	Duration
Fast-acting: Lispro (Humalog) Aspart (Novolog) Glulisine (Apidra)	5–15 minutes	45–75 minutes	2–4 hours
Regular	20–30 minutes	2–4 hours	5–8 hours
70/30	30–60 minutes	3–8 hours	12–18 hours
NPH	About 2 hours	6–10 hours	12–18 hours
Long-acting: Glargine (Lantus) Detemir (Levemir)	About 2 hours	Small peak at no predictable time	18–24 hours

Why should I take more than one type of insulin?

You may not need to, but most people do better on both a long-acting insulin and a fast-acting insulin. Whether you have diabetes or not, you need some insulin in your body at all times. Even between meals or when you are fasting or sleeping, your body needs a small, steady amount of insulin around to help your brain, muscles, and other organs use glucose and function properly. This low, flat trickle of insulin is sometimes called the basal insulin. But whenever you eat food, especially carbohydrates, you need much more insulin for the next few hours to help you deal with that food to move the glucose and fat out of your blood into your cells. This is sometimes called an insulin spike, or a bolus. You may need one or two shots of a long-acting insulin and two or three shots of a fast-acting insulin to cover the food you eat at your main meals.

Exactly how much insulin, how many shots, and what types are best for you is something for you to talk to your doctor about. In the answers to the next several questions, I will try to explain some of the things for you to think about that will help you have a more informed conversation with your doctor.

How high a dose of insulin can you give?

A healthy, non-diabetic person who weighs 154 pounds (70 kilograms) produces 30–60 units of insulin from his or her pancreas every day. Someone who is much heavier will be more resistant to insulin and could easily make four times as much. If you have diabetes, how much insulin you need depends on how much insulin (if any) you make yourself and how resistant to the effects of insulin you are. In general people who are overweight or obese need more insulin than people who are lean, but there is a huge range in the insulin dose that people need. If you take ten people with type 1 diabetes who all weigh 200 lbs (91 kg), the amount of insulin that they need could vary enormously. There is really no upper limit to the dose of insulin.

In the past thirty years, I have had a handful of patients who have needed over 2000 units of insulin per day. They have a rare condition called partial lipodystrophy, where they have almost no subcutaneous body fat and yet are extremely resistant to insulin. I had to talk to the insulin manufacturers to get a supply of specially made, concentrated insulin, just so that my patients wouldn't have to inject such a large volume under their skin. Most insulin comes with 100 units in every cubic centimeter (cc) or milliliter (ml). So if you are taking 20 units at a time, this is a small volume to inject (0.2 ml). But if you have to take 500 units three or four times a day, that would be 5 ml of liquid to inject. For those rare patients, it is possible to get insulin that contains 500 units in every milliliter.

Most people with diabetes need less than 100 units of insulin a day, but I have many patients (usually people who have type 2 diabetes and who are overweight) who need 200–400 units a day. If you need a higher dose of insulin than other people, this doesn't mean that your diabetes is "worse" than theirs or "more severe" than theirs. It simply means that you either make less insulin than they do or you are more insulin resistant than they are. How healthy you stay over the years has very little to do with how much insulin you need to take. It has far more to do with how well you can control your blood glucose, your blood pressure, your cholesterol, and your lifestyle.

How can I decide what the best types of insulin are for me?

This is something you really need to talk to your doctor about. It depends on what type of diabetes you have, how complicated your lifestyle is, what other illnesses you have to deal with, and how much money you can afford to pay. The newer insulins are more expensive. Although they offer some advantages, if money is a significant barrier to you, it is possible to get quite good control of your blood glucose with the older and cheaper insulins like Regular and NPH.

What are the differences between the fast-acting insulins?

All three of the fast-acting insulin analogs have almost identical profiles when they are injected. They all "kick in" (or have their onset) within five to fifteen minutes and have their peak effect about forty-five to seventy-five minutes later. They all "run out" about two to four hours after you inject them. There are very tiny differences between them. Some people with diabetes who have used one brand of fast-acting insulin for years will complain when they are switched to another brand. I have had heated conversations from patients who were switched from Humalog to Novolog and are sure that the Humalog worked better. I don't argue with them. They may be right, or they may just feel more comfortable with an insulin they are familiar with. When scientists have injected the same amount of Humalog, Novolog, or Apidra into a few dozen research volunteers, using carefully controlled conditions, and have measured how fast the insulin rises, when it peaks, and how long it lasts, the results are almost identical.

How soon before a meal should I inject my fast-acting insulin?

If you are using Humalog, Novolog, or Apidra, it is best to inject it immediately before you start eating. You should not give yourself the injection until the food is on the table in front of you. I have had patients tell me stories of eating out at a restaurant where they ordered their meal and expected it to arrive within five minutes. They went to the restroom to check their blood glucose and gave themselves their shot of Humalog or Novolog before returning to their table. After ten or fifteen minutes, the waiter came back and apologized that they were out of some critical ingredient, or a new chef had burnt it, or a new waiter had dropped their order on the floor! Those patients then described feeling their blood glucose dropping and frantically eating bread or crackers to stop themselves passing out from hypoglycemia before their meal arrived. If you are eating at home, you have more control over when the food will arrive, but even there you can run into problems.

Let's say you check your blood glucose, give yourself your insulin shot, and then start to make your meal. Maybe you already have the pasta pot boiling. When you open the cupboard, you suddenly realize you are out of pasta. Or the phone rings, and it is your best friend. You haven't talked to her in ages, and before you know it, you are deep in conversation. You weren't that hungry anyway. But five or ten minutes later, you suddenly feel sweaty and shaky and start slurring your speech. Your friend says, "Are you okay? You sound weird. Is your sugar getting too low?"

As with all "rules," you can decide for yourself how and when to bend or break them. You will get used to how quickly your fast-acting insulin seems to "kick in" for you. If your blood glucose before the meal is high, then you will be safer taking the insulin shot further ahead of the meal than if your blood glucose is already low. But the safest thing to do is to wait until the food is right there in front of you before you give yourself your shot of fast-acting insulin.

How do you decide how much fast-acting insulin to give before a meal?

There are different ways to figure this out. You should discuss the options with your doctor. The simplest approach is to always eat the same amount of carbohydrate at each meal and always give the same dose of fast-acting insulin. I have some patients who say that they don't want to have to think and they don't want to have to check their blood glucose before every meal, so they always eat 60 grams of carbohydrate and always give themselves the same dose of fast-acting insulin. I don't like this approach. It is not a good idea to give yourself a shot of fast-acting insulin before a meal if you don't know what your blood glucose is at the time. Even if you have the same amount of carbohydrate at every meal and know that 6 units of Apidra or Novolog should "cover" that amount of carbohydrate, you might need more than 6 units.

If your blood glucose before the start of the meal is already much higher than usual, you should take more than your usual six units. And if your blood glucose is really low before the start of the meal, you might do better by taking less. So you might work out with your doctor a "sliding scale." This means that you vary the dose of fast-acting insulin depending on what your blood glucose is. It might say:

Example only

Blood glucose	Insulin dose
Less than 100	Take no insulin
100–150	6
151–200	8
201–250	10
Over 250	12

Let me be clear. DO NOT start using this sliding scale. I am giving it as an example. Exactly how much insulin you need before a meal will vary tremendously from one person to the next. You need to discuss it with your own doctor. The most sophisticated way to decide how much fast-acting insulin to take before a meal is to vary it depending on both what your blood glucose is immediately before the meal and also how much carbohydrate you are going to eat.

Here is another example of pre-meal instructions that I might give to guide one of my patients:

For your basic dose take 1 unit of insulin to cover every 15 grams of carbohydrate.

- If your blood glucose is 70–130, take the basic dose only.
- If your blood glucose is 131–160, take the basic dose plus 1.
- If your blood glucose is 161–190, take the basic dose plus 2.
- If your blood glucose is 191–220, take the basic dose plus 3.
- If your blood glucose is 221–250, take the basic dose plus 4.

I might also add a line that says, "If your blood glucose is less than 70 before you start the meal, go ahead and eat the meal and take 2 units less than your basic dose, and take it at the end of the meal.

Again, please DO NOT follow these instructions without talking to your own doctor. Some people need much more or less insulin than others.

Isn't if better to give the insulin after the meal, when you know how high the blood glucose has gone?

Although that sounds sensible, there are a couple of reasons why it is not a good approach. How high your blood glucose goes after a meal depends on how long after the meal you tested, how much carbohydrate was in the meal, how much protein and fat was in the meal, how much insulin you already have in your body, and whether your insulin level is rising or falling. Let me give you a couple of really different examples.

Let's say you just ate a white bread sandwich with a thick layer of jam on it and washed it down with a large glass of regular pop. If you checked your blood glucose thirty minutes after that meal, you would be shocked at how high it was. That meal is made almost entirely of "simple" (or refined) carbohydrate. Your body absorbs it very quickly, so your blood glucose goes up very fast. If you measured your blood glucose one or two hours after the meal, you would probably get a much lower reading. So the dose of insulin you took would vary depending on when you tested. If you overreacted to the high blood glucose reading at thirty minutes, you might take too much insulin and push your blood glucose down to hypoglycemic levels an hour later.

Take another example. Let's say you ate a large helping of pizza covered in cheese and pepperoni. Even though there is a lot of carbohydrate in that meal, the fat and protein in it would slow down the rate at which the food leaves your stomach and gets absorbed. So if you measured your blood glucose one hour after the meal, it might not seem all that high; and so you might give yourself too little insulin, and so your blood glucose would still be high a few hours later.

Is it ever okay to inject insulin after the meal?

Yes. There are a couple of situations when this is a good idea. If your blood glucose is already low before the start of the meal and you are feeling hypoglycemic, it makes sense to go ahead and start eating, and then take your fast-acting insulin at the end of the meal. I also advise the moms and dads of diabetic toddlers to wait to the end of the meal before they decide how much insulin to give. Let's say that little Johnny, an adorable but spirited two-year-old, has diabetes and needs 1 unit of fast-acting insulin to cover every 30 grams of carbohydrate that he eats. Mom checks his blood glucose before the meal and serves Johnny a plate of noodles and a glass of milk that she estimates contains a total of 90 grams of carbohydrate. She gives Johnny his insulin and then puts the meal in front of him. If Johnny pours the milk on top of the noodles or tips it onto the floor and then has tantrums and decides he won't eat it, then Mom has a problem. Johnny is going to become hypoglycemic unless Mom can persuade him to eat something else with enough carbohydrate in it to cover the amount of insulin that is already in his body from the shot of fast-acting insulin.

A better approach might be to check the blood glucose before the meal, serve Johnny his food, and estimate how much he actually eats. Then, just before he leaves the table, Mom can give him enough insulin to cover the amount of carbohydrate he actually ate, plus enough to adjust for what his blood glucose was before the meal. I have some adult patients who confess that they have as little willpower as a toddler! They say that they never know how much carbohydrate they are going to eat, so they wait until the end of the meal to give themselves a dose. I must say patients who do this very rarely have good blood glucose control.

What are the differences between the longer-acting insulins?

They vary in how long they last, how much of a peak they have, and when that peak occurs. The ranges that I gave in the table on page 244 are only an approximate guide. There is a big difference from one person to the next. Most people who take NPH insulin notice that it gives them a peak about six or eight hours after they take it and that the effect of any shot of NPH has mostly worn off by about twelve hours. Because of that, they need to make sure they have something to eat six or eight hours after they have taken it. They also need to take two shots a day. Some people like that peak. If they take NPH insulin in the morning before they leave for work, the peak of the NPH occurs in the middle of the day when they are going to eat lunch anyway. So they don't need to give themselves a shot of fast-acting insulin before lunch. I have other patients who tell me that a single dose of NPH in the morning will last them all the way through to the next morning. That is uncommon but does occur.

Both Lantus and Levemir last longer than NPH. They also have smaller peaks. The drug companies that make these insulins like to advertise them as having no peak, but that is not always true. They also like to claim that these insulins last for a full twenty-four hours on a single shot. This is sometimes true, but not always.

How do you choose the right size of insulin syringe and needle?

To choose the right size of syringe, it depends on how big a dose of insulin you take at any one shot. Insulin syringes come in sizes that take up to 30 units, 50 units, or 100 units of insulin. Insulin pens can dial up to 70 units in a single shot. When choosing a needle, you need to think about the length and thickness of the needle. If you are a thin person, you do not want to use a needle that is too long, or it may go through the fat under your skin and into the muscle underneath. That would result in a more painful injection and would make the insulin be absorbed much more quickly, putting you at risk of hypoglycemia. But if you have thick skin and use a needle that is too short, it may not get all the way through into the subcutaneous fat. This could result in a painful injection where the insulin is not well absorbed.

When looking at how thin a needle is, the higher the "gauge," the thinner it is, so a 29G needle is thinner than a 27G needle. The thinner the needle, the less painful the shot will be. However, if you are using cloudy insulin (like NPH), it can sometimes be difficult to push through the very fine needles. I usually start my patients out with a 31G needle that is three-eighths of an inch long and adjust from there.

Should my spouse or close friend know how to give me my shot?

This is up to you, but there are few reasons why someone else would need to give you an insulin shot. If you have arthritis in your hands or your hand trembles too much to hold steady, or if you can't see well enough to draw up the correct dose, then your partner or close friend can be shown how to give your shot. Some people find it really difficult to give themselves a shot in the arm, and so they have someone else do it for them. But for most people, you feel much more independent and flexible if you give your own shots.

How often should I change the needle on my syringe or pen?

The manufacturers say that you should change the needle for every injection that you give. In truth you can use the same needle two or three times before changing it, so long as it is only you who uses that needle and so long as it doesn't feel clogged up or blunt. Some of the newer insulin needles are extremely thin. This makes them less painful when you stick yourself, but also makes them bend or clog more easily. But if you are careful with your needle and it doesn't feel bent, blunt, or clogged when you use it a second or third time, it is quite safe to do so. If you use your insulin pen to give your fast-acting insulin before breakfast, lunch, and dinner every day, then putting a fresh needle on each morning is a good idea. If you prefer to change the needle every time, that is fine, but it is probably not necessary. You can discuss this with your own doctor.

Should I swab my skin with alcohol before injecting myself?

There is no need to do this. Swabbing your skin with alcohol is likely to make your skin tougher and may also make the injection sting more than if you don't use alcohol. Insulin, and the preservatives that are in the bottle or cartridge, is sterile when you get it and is not a place where bacteria are likely to grow. It is incredibly rare for people who inject themselves with insulin to get skin infections at the site where they inject. There is also no scientific evidence that swabbing the skin with alcohol before giving your injection makes infection less likely.

I think it is safe and sensible to give your injections directly into clean, dry skin. You should wash your hands before you inject and should be very careful to keep the needle covered before and after giving yourself a shot.

Where is the best place on my body to inject insulin?

Insulin is absorbed well from the layer of fat that lies under your skin. All of the estimates of the onset, peak, and duration of a particular type of insulin assume that the insulin was injected into this layer of fat under the skin. If you injected too deeply by mistake and the insulin went into a muscle that was under the skin, then the insulin would be absorbed much faster. This is most likely to happen if you do not have much fat covering the muscles on part of your leg. Muscles have a bigger supply of blood vessels running through them, and so injecting into a muscle is more likely to bleed. It also makes it more likely that you will have a low blood glucose level in the next hour or two.

So make sure there is a layer of fat below the skin where you are injecting.

The most common sites to inject are the abdomen, the thigh, the buttocks, and the upper arm. Some people find that the skin over their abdomen is a bit more tender than the skin on those other places. There is also a layer of fibrous tissue running up and down in the middle of your abdomen (above and below your belly button), so you should avoid that part. Insulin is absorbed slightly faster from the abdomen and slower from the buttocks and thighs (with the arm being in between). So if you find that your long-acting insulin is not lasting long enough when you give the injection in your abdomen, then switching to give it in your buttock might work better.

What is the best system for rotating my insulin shots?

You will hear all sorts of ideas for how to do this. Some diabetes instruction manuals show a diagram of the body with areas marked out like a tic-tac-toe grid on your abdomen, thighs, and upper arm. I have seen some patients who took that advice literally and marked grids on their skin with felt tip pens to keep track of where they should inject next! Some people stick to one place for a week and then move to another part of their body. The problem with that approach is that insulin is absorbed at different rates from different places. So if you gave all your shots in your buttock or thigh for a week and then moved to your abdomen, you might notice that your blood glucose readings were different.

A system that works well for a lot of people is to take your long-acting insulin in your buttock or thigh and your fast-acting pre-meal shots in your abdomen. You want the long-acting insulin to be absorbed slowly and the fast-acting insulin to be absorbed fast, so injecting in those areas makes sense. Besides, it is easier to inject in your buttock or thigh when you are at home, and it is easier to inject in the abdomen when you are out in public. So long as you move around and use different places for your shots, you should be able to come up with a system that suits you.

Chapter 26

Insulin Management

- Why can I give the same dose of the same insulin two days in a row and get completely different blood glucose results?
- What things affect insulin absorption?
- Is it best to give the long-acting insulin in the morning or at night?
- Isn't there insulin that lasts for twenty-four hours nowadays?
- How would I know if my long-acting insulin is lasting for twenty-four hours?
- What is the Somogyi phenomenon?
- When is it okay to use only one type of insulin?
- What are the advantages of mixing different types of insulin together?
- What are the disadvantages of mixing different types of insulin together?
- Is it better to use a syringe or an insulin pen?
- How long does a bottle of insulin last once it is opened?
- If I find a spot where it doesn't hurt so much, why can't I inject there all the time?
- What should I do if I take too much insulin by accident?
- What should I do if I forget to take an insulin shot?
- What is "brittle diabetes"?
- Is there damage from long term insulin use?

Why can I give the same dose of the same insulin two days in a row and get completely different blood glucose results?

One reason is that insulin is absorbed at different rates from different parts of your body. If you inject into a part of your body where there wasn't much fat and so the needle went right into muscle (this is particularly likely when you inject in some parts of your leg), the insulin will be absorbed much faster. If you inject into a scarred area, then the insulin will be absorbed slower. Even if you inject into the fat under your skin, it will be absorbed faster if you inject into your abdomen, a bit slower if you inject into your arm, and slower still if you inject into your buttocks or thighs. Even if you inject in the same part of your body on those two days, you might still get different blood glucose results a few hours later. There might be differences in how many blood vessels were near the injection. It might be warmer on one day and colder on the other day, and that could affect how much blood was flowing near the injection.

I don't want you to think that the situation is hopeless, but the truth is that injecting a drug or hormone under the skin is a fairly crude (or imprecise) way of delivering that drug or hormone. The amount of insulin that is in your blood six hours after injecting the same dose of insulin on two different days can actually vary by 30 percent or more.

What things affect insulin absorption?

The bigger the dose of insulin you take, the more the absorption will vary from one day to the next. If you need to inject more than 50 units as a single dose, then you often get more predictable absorption if you split it into two smaller shots injected into two different places. I saw a patient recently who was taking 140 units of NPH insulin twice a day and still had really high blood glucose levels. She had an insulin pen that could be dialed up to 70 units at a time. She would dial it up to 70, inject that under her skin, and then dial it up to 70 again (without taking the needle out) and inject another 70 right in the same spot. So she had 140 units all "slopped together" in the same place under her skin. I told her to reduce her dose to 90 units but take it as three separate shots of 30 units each time. To her surprise, her blood glucose levels got lower, even though she seemed to be taking less insulin. The explanation is that a lot of the insulin from her big 140-unit shot was not getting into her blood, but when she took three smaller shots, the insulin absorption was improved. Please do not try doing this on your own.

Talk to your doctor about it before you make any changes. The variation in insulin absorption is worse with long-acting insulin than with fast-acting insulin. So it is worse with NPH than with Regular, Humalog, Novolog, or Apidra. Among the long-acting insulins, it is worse with NPH than with Lantus. Levemir seems to cause the least variation in absorption of all the long-acting insulins.

Is it best to give the long-acting insulin in the morning or at night?

It really depends on what the rest of your life is like. For most people with type 1 diabetes, taking the long acting insulin in the morning is the first thing to try. Obviously if you work a night shift, then you may need to think differently, but when you get up for the day and are about to have breakfast, then that is a good time to take a long-acting insulin to give you some "background" or "basal" insulin during the day. But like so many things about managing your diabetes, the real answer is to try it one way for a while, check your blood glucose levels, check how you feel, and then decide if it is working or if you should try something different. You might do great taking a single shot of long-acting insulin in the morning; you might do better taking it at night; or you might need to take your long-acting insulin twice a day.

Isn't there insulin that lasts for twenty-four hours nowadays?

The pharmaceutical companies who make Lantus and Levemir insulin would like you to believe that their insulin lasts for twenty-four hours on a single daily injection. One of the compelling ads for Lantus shows a neon motel sign lit up at nighttime, saying "Open 24 hours." It is an appealing idea: you just need to give one shot a day and get a nice, steady, predictable, flat, basal insulin delivery for the next twenty-four hours. The truth is that while Lantus and Levemir sometimes work like that, there are other times when these insulins last less than twenty-four hours, and so you have to take two shots a day.

How would I know if my long-acting insulin is lasting for twenty-four hours?

Let's say you take your Lantus or Levemir first thing in the morning, after you have slept for eight hours and before you have eaten anything. Your average fasting blood glucose is too high (let's say 180 mg/dL, or 10 mmol/L). Your doctor will probably advise you to increase the dose of your Lantus or Levemir insulin. If you increase by a few units every week and your fasting blood glucose average over the next several weeks comes down steadily until it is at 120 mg/dL and you feel fine, then your long-acting insulin is probably lasting for twenty-four hours. However, if you start increasing your morning dose of Lantus or Levemir and your fasting blood glucose average stays too high, there might be a problem.

If you keep increasing a few units a week but now you find your blood glucose is dropping too low during the afternoon or evening—and your fasting blood glucose is still too high—then that probably means that your long-acting insulin is running out before the twenty-four hours is up. Maybe it is only lasting about twenty hours, but for the last few hours of the night, while you are asleep, you have too little insulin in your body; and so your liver pushes out glucose, and you wake up with a blood glucose that is too high.

In that situation you might do better splitting your Lantus or Levemir dose into two equal halves and taking them about twelve hours apart. Each dose will last about twenty hours, but the doses will overlap and give you a much more stable basal insulin level. I find that I need to do this about a third of the time with my patients who have type 1 diabetes. It is something to talk to your doctor about if you can't keep your fasting blood glucose in a good range with just one shot a day of your long-acting insulin.

What is the Somogyi phenomenon?

In the 1930s Michael Somogyi suggested that when someone with diabetes takes too much insulin and becomes hypoglycemic, this causes an excessive release of other hormones (like adrenaline, glucagon, growth hormone, and cortisol), resulting in an exaggerated "rebound hyperglycemia." So if you wake up with a high blood glucose, the theory says it was because you went too low in the middle of the night and got "rebound hyperglycemia" because of an exaggerated release of hormones that squeezed lots and lots of glucose out of your liver to compensate for the hypoglycemia.

Despite the fact that careful scientific studies have repeatedly shown that Somogyi was wrong, this idea of "rebound hyperglycemia" has persisted in the medical literature for almost a century. A Google search turns up over a million responses, including articles talking about how to recognize the Somogyi phenomenon in your pets! I have three theories about why this myth persists. First, the phrase just sounds nice. I have heard doctors or the parents of diabetic children turn Somogyi's name into a verb. "Little Johnny was cranky this morning. He must have been Somogying last night." Second, it is appealing because it is quirky and counterintuitive. Somogyi actually suggested that if you wake up with your blood glucose too high, it is because you had too much insulin the previous night, and you need to decrease it rather than increase it to "fix" the problem. Third, Somogyi understood part of the problem, and so his theory sounds possible.

If Somogyi was correct, then the lower your blood glucose went during the night, the higher it would be in the morning. Just the opposite is true. He suggested that if you reduce your evening insulin, you will go less low during the night and so will wake up with a better (lower) glucose in the morning. This is also not true. If you lower your evening insulin enough, you can certainly get rid of the overnight low blood glucose, but your morning blood glucose will be worse (higher), not better. The most common reason that people with diabetes go too low during the night is that they have too much insulin in their blood at that time.

I see it most often when people are taking NPH insulin (or one of the 70/30 insulin mixtures) before their evening meal. The insulin peaks in the middle of the night and causes severe hypoglycemia at 1:00 or 2:00 a.m. The insulin then runs out sometime between 3:00 and 8:00 a.m., so their blood glucose rises rapidly. (If there isn't enough insulin in your blood, then the liver releases a lot of glucose into your blood.) The way to fix the problem is NOT to decrease the dose of NPH or 70/30 insulin. The best solution is to switch to a type of insulin that has less of a peak during the middle of the night but lasts long enough so that it doesn't run out before the morning.

When is it okay to use only one type of insulin?

This does not often work well if you have type 1 diabetes. Human beings need a flat basal amount of insulin when they are fasting or sleeping but need spikes of higher amounts of fast-acting insulin for a few hours after meals. If you have type 1 diabetes and make no insulin of your own, then you will almost certainly do better taking shots of a long-acting insulin and shots of fast-acting insulin to cover your meals. I have some very old patients who are either too forgetful or too stiff and sore to give their own insulin injections. If they stop insulin altogether, their blood glucose is too high and they feel miserable, but no one is around during the day to give them shots of fast-acting insulin before their meals. If someone can come in once a day in the morning and give them a shot of long-acting insulin, they feel a whole lot better. This is a compromise. They don't have great blood glucose control (as measured by their HbA1c level), but they have a decent quality of life, because they are not thirsty and tired and going to the bathroom all of the time.

What are the advantages of mixing different types of insulin together?

It is appealing to just take one shot in the morning and then forget about your diabetes for the rest of the day. Many pediatricians (doctors who look after children) used to give a once a day cocktail of two, three, or even four different types of insulin as a single shot in the morning. The syringe would contain some fast-acting insulin to cover breakfast, a medium-acting insulin like NPH to cover the middle of the day, and a very long-acting insulin to cover the evening and overnight.

A more common approach that I still see used a lot is for people to take an insulin that has fast-acting and medium-acting insulin mixed together so that they only need to take two shots a day. Seventy/thirty insulin contains 70 percent NPH and 30 percent Regular. There is also a 50/50 mixture of NPH and Regular and a 75/25 mixture of Humalog and a longer-acting insulin. Nobody enjoys giving themselves injections, so fewer insulin shots seems like a good idea. If both you and your doctor believe that these "pre-mixed" insulins give an early peak from the fast-acting insulin and then a later peak or a flatter basal amount of insulin a few hours later, all from a single shot, what's not to like about that?

What are the disadvantages of mixing different types of insulin together?

The problem with mixing fast-acting insulin along with medium or long-acting insulin is that you don't get two separate peaks. If you think about it, this is not surprising. NPH insulin is basically Regular insulin with stuff added to the bottle to slow it down. The "stuff" is a fish protein called protamine, along with some zinc and other preservatives. If you add more Regular insulin to the mixture, then that insulin will get slowed down, too.

If you add in the problem that the absorption of all of these insulins is rather variable from day to day, you can imagine why so few people get great blood glucose control by using pre-mixed insulins. They give unpredictable single peaks sometime between three and eight hours after you take the shot. Unless you can recognize your symptoms of hypoglycemia and can eat enough carbohydrate to treat it, you are likely to find that taking a pre-mixed insulin does not give you great blood glucose control.

Is it better to use a syringe or an insulin pen?

A bottle of insulin contains 10 ml of liquid with 1000 units of insulin in it. Insulin pens contain cartridges of 3 ml, or 300 units of insulin. Some pens are prefilled. You just throw the pen away (in a disposable "Sharps" container) when you have used up all the insulin. Other pens come with replaceable cartridges so that you only throw away the used cartridge when it is empty. You keep the pen and put in a new cartridge.

The biggest advantage of using an insulin pen is convenience. This is especially true if you take fast-acting insulin before every meal. During the day or when you are eating out, it is much easier to take an insulin pen with you to give that pre-meal shot of insulin instead of having to take your insulin bottle, some alcohol swabs (to clean the rubber covering on the bottle), and a syringe and needle to draw up your insulin. Another advantage of insulin pens is that if you only take a small dose (6 units or less), then they give a more accurate dose than drawing insulin out of a bottle into a syringe.

The main disadvantage of insulin pens is that they are more expensive, although that is changing as they become more and more widely used. Another thing to be careful about is keeping the insulin cool. All insulin, whether it is in a pen or in a bottle, can be damaged if it is left in a hot environment. So if you leave your insulin pen in your purse lying on the front seat of your car in scorching hot weather for hours on end, then the insulin might get "cooked" and lose its potency. While this is true for any insulin, it is more likely to be a problem with an insulin pen.

If you get a box of three or four disposable insulin pens, you should store the unused pens in your refrigerator, but you can take the pen you are using with you in your jacket or your purse. As long as it stays cool and you use up the insulin in the pen within two or three weeks, it should work just fine. But if you leave your insulin pen lying above a radiator or on the dashboard of your car baking in the sun, then the insulin is not likely to work the way you expect.

How long does a bottle of insulin last once it is opened?

This depends on a lot of things, especially the temperature that the insulin is kept at. A good general rule is that if the bottle is being kept in the refrigerator, it will last four weeks after it has been opened. You should start a new bottle after four weeks, even if there is still some insulin left in it. If the insulin is kept out of the refrigerator after it has been opened, it will last for at least two weeks if it is kept cool, but you should consider starting a new bottle (or a new cartridge or pen) after two weeks.

If I find a spot where it doesn't hurt so much, why can't I inject there all the time?

This is not a good idea. When you inject into the fat under your skin, that insulin sits there for hours on end and gradually gets absorbed into your blood. While it is sitting there, the insulin stimulates the fat cells nearby, and they swell a little as they take up more glucose and turn that into fat. If you move your injection around and don't come back to the same spot for several days, this is not a problem. But if you keep injecting into the very same small area every day, then two things happen. The local fat swells more and more until you may have a noticeable blubbery lump on that part of your body. The medical term for this is lipohypertrophy (which is just Latin for "fat enlargement"). This can look odd, especially if it is on part of your body that other people can see (like the upper arm or your legs during the summer). Also, the insulin that you inject into those lumpy areas does not get absorbed into your blood very well, and so you need to give bigger and bigger doses to get your blood glucose to come down.

What should I do if I take too much insulin by accident?

It depends on how much extra insulin you gave and what type of insulin it was. I had a patient who was supposed to take 4 units of fast-acting Novolog insulin before her breakfast and 36 units of Novolin NPH insulin. She got them mixed up and gave herself 36 units of the fast-acting Novolog by mistake. Because Novolog is a very fast-acting insulin that has its peak effect about an hour after you inject it and lasts about three hours altogether, I told her to stay home, eat lots of extra carbohydrate, and test her blood glucose every fifteen minutes for the next four hours. If you inject too much of a long-acting insulin, then you will need to keep testing your blood glucose for much longer and be prepared to take extra carbohydrate food for several hours until the extra insulin has worn off.

What should I do if I forget to take an insulin shot?

It depends what type of insulin you forgot to take. If you sat down to eat a meal and realized an hour after the meal that you had forgotten to take your dose of fast-acting insulin before the meal, it would be a good idea to take some of your fast-acting insulin right then. If you remember immediately after the meal, then you should probably take your usual pre-meal dose. If you only remember one or two hours after the meal, I would recommend that you only take about half your usual pre-meal dose, and if it is three or more hours after the meal, you should probably just wait until the next meal before you take any more insulin.

If it is your long-acting insulin that you forget, then what to do depends on how big a dose of insulin you missed, what type of insulin it was, and how long after you should have taken it you remember. You should certainly check your blood glucose and figure out when your next dose would be due. Sometimes taking a partial dose makes sense, but if you are hours overdue, it might be best to wait until your next dose is due. Taking extra doses of insulin at unusual times in between your usual doses can result in "stacking" of the insulin effect. If you usually take a dose of NPH insulin every twelve hours, for example, but forget a dose and then take it six hours late, this means that when you take your next dose at the proper time, you will still have a lot of insulin in your body from the extra dose, and the effect of this will be "stacked" on top of your usual dose—putting you at increased risk of a low blood glucose. Because there are so many variables to think about, this is a situation when it is best to check your blood glucose frequently and, if possible, check in with your own doctor for specific advice.

What is "brittle diabetes"?

If you have diabetes, I am sure you have noticed that your blood glucose sometimes swings from high levels to low levels for no apparent reason. You scratch your head and adjust what you are eating or what you are doing or take an extra dose of insulin, but you can't think why your blood glucose was so high or so low at that particular moment. These unpredictable swings in blood glucose can be so severe and frequent that it makes your life miserable.

Professor Robert Tattersall of the University of Nottingham in England came up with the term *brittle diabetes* to describe "the patient whose life is constantly disrupted by episodes of hyper- or hypoglycemia, whatever their cause." People with brittle diabetes may have to be admitted to hospital several times a year because of severe hypoglycemia or because of diabetic ketoacidosis. Usually they have a lot of stress and unhappiness in their life so that they just can't focus on all the things that they need to do to keep their diabetes under reasonable control. It is most common to see brittle diabetes in teenagers and young adults. Once their lives get sorted out and they become happier and more stable, then their diabetes becomes a lot less brittle.

Is there damage from long term insulin use?

Some people worry that giving all of these shots of insulin under the skin will cause so much scarring that they will run out of places to inject. That never happens. I have several patients who have been injecting themselves with insulin several times a day for over fifty years and have no problems finding places to inject themselves. Although insulin injections can sometimes cause bruising or lumps to form at the place where you inject, these quickly heal up.

Another worry is that the high level of insulin in your blood from all of these injections might make you more likely to deposit fat in the lining of your blood vessels and so increase your risk of heart attacks or strokes. Several large research studies have shown that this is not true. By far the biggest risk to your health if you have diabetes is for your blood glucose to be too high for years on end. If you are doing the best you can to eat healthy and get exercise and are taking pills for diabetes, but your blood glucose is still too high, then taking insulin to bring your blood glucose down is a far healthier and better decision to make than to avoid taking insulin because you think the insulin might cause damage to your body.

Chapter 27

Advanced Insulin Management

- Isn't it easier to use an insulin pump?
- What are the advantages of an insulin pump?
- What are the disadvantages of an insulin pump?
- How good is inhaled insulin?
- How does pramlintide (Symlin) work?
- What are the benefits of using pramlintide (Symlin)?
- What are the problems with pramlintide (Symlin)?

Isn't it easier to use an insulin pump?

Insulin pumps can be a great way to manage type 1 diabetes for some people, but I doubt if many of them would say it is easy. Remember, an insulin pump doesn't measure your blood glucose. It doesn't automatically change how much insulin it gives you until you tell it to. It won't stop giving you insulin just because your blood glucose is too low or give you more when your glucose is too high. It is a complicated and expensive piece of technology and comes with a lot of supplies to learn about and keep track of. If it breaks down and stops working, you would be in trouble in a few hours, and so most people who use an insulin pump also keep some fast-acting and long-acting insulin, syringes, or pens as a backup.

What are the advantages of an insulin pump?

The biggest advantage that an insulin pump gives is a very steady and predictable basal insulin rate. Let's say that you are taking 24 units of Lantus insulin once a day in the morning. That large collection of long-acting insulin is supposed to be slowly released from the fat under your skin to give you about 1 unit of insulin per hour. But a lot of factors affect how well that insulin is released. There is a lot of day-to-day variation. If I was to measure the insulin level in your blood at 11:00 a.m. every day, five hours after you took that 24 units of Lantus, it might vary by 30 percent or more from day to day. The same is true for most other long-acting insulin. But with a pump, you do not have a large collection of insulin under your skin. The pump trickles in a tiny amount of fast-acting insulin all the time, and it is absorbed into your blood almost immediately. To give you the same amount of insulin as that 24 units of Lantus, the pump gives a tenth of a unit of insulin every six minutes to give you 1 unit per hour. If I measured the insulin level in your blood at 11:00 a.m. every day, there would be hardly any variation from one day to the next.

Another advantage with a pump is that you can program it to increase that basal rate during the night while you are sleeping. Some people wake up with higher blood glucose readings in the morning because of the dawn phenomenon. In the few hours before you wake up, your body pushes out a lot of cortisol and growth hormone. These make you more insulin resistant, and so your blood glucose will rise, unless you can increase the amount of insulin in your blood during those hours. If that is a problem for you, then an insulin pump can help by stepping up your basal insulin rate while you sleep. You don't have to stick yourself so many times with syringes or insulin pens if you are on a pump. Instead, once every three days you stick yourself with a needle and then leave a small, thin plastic tube under the skin to deliver insulin. Some people find this to be a lot more comfortable.

What are the disadvantages of an insulin pump?

Insulin pumps are expensive. The cost to you will depend on what insurance coverage you have; but most pumps are four or five thousand dollars to purchase, and the supplies can be another couple of hundred dollars every month. You still have to prick your finger several times a day and then tell the pump how much fast-acting insulin to push in before each meal. You are wearing a device about the size of a cell phone that is attached to you all the time. You can take it off for an hour at a time if you are having a shower, swimming, or being intimate, but the rest of the time, you need to keep your pump attached to you. Some people don't mind that. It drives other people nuts.

You can find out a lot more at the American Diabetes Association website at http://www.diabetes.org/type-1-diabetes/insulin-pumps.jsp. Several good, practical books have been written that can give you a better idea if an insulin pump would be good for you or not. I like *Smart Pumping* by Howard Wolpert, MD, but there are many others.

How good is inhaled insulin?

A lot of people like the idea of inhaled insulin, because it would be less painful to suck in a dose of insulin instead of sticking yourself and injecting it under the skin. Insulin is absorbed quite fast once it gets to the warm, wet, spongy tissue of your lungs. But there are several practical problems and concerns about using inhaled insulin. You will still need to take one or two shots of a long-acting insulin every day. Inhaled insulin would only replace your pre-meal fast-acting insulin. You need to take a much bigger dose of insulin if you are inhaling it, because about 90 percent of it gets stuck in your mouth and throat and never reaches your lungs.

Several companies are working on inhaled insulin. Some of them use powdered insulin that is packaged into little capsules. You insert a capsule into a device that looks a bit like an asthma inhaler, puncture the capsule, and then suck it into your lungs. It is very difficult to adjust the dose of insulin using a system like this. You can't make the kind of precise variations in dose that you can with an insulin pen or a syringe. I have a few patients who are using inhaled insulin as part of research studies. After a year, they are having just as much hypoglycemia as they were before, and their HbA1c is the same or slightly higher. None of them feel that it has made their life better or easier. The first pharmaceutical company to put inhaled insulin on the market was Pfizer. They called their inhaled insulin Exubera. It has not caught on in popularity, and in 2007 Pfizer took it off the market.

There are some other concerns with inhaled insulin. People who use inhaled insulin tend to develop insulin antibodies more often than those who inject it under their skin. When we measure how well their lungs are able to diffuse oxygen, this also gets a little worse. Scientists do not know whether either of these things will cause long-term problems or not. You will probably hear a lot more about inhaled insulin over the next few years.

How does pramlintide (Symlin) work?

The islet cells in a healthy pancreas not only make insulin to push out into the blood, they also make another hormone called amylin. Amylin is pushed out along with insulin after a meal. It slows stomach emptying and helps make you feel full and satisfied after eating. It also stops your body pushing out too much of another hormone called glucagon. By doing all of those things, amylin helps the blood glucose to rise more slowly after a meal. Because the islet cells get destroyed if you have type 1 diabetes, you stop making amylin as well as insulin. Although amylin can be manufactured and given back to people who don't make it anymore, it is very quickly broken down in the body and so only works if it is given continuously. Pramlintide (Symlin) is a synthetic long-acting form of amylin that can be given as an injection under the skin before each meal.

What are the benefits of using pramlintide (Symlin)?

Like so many new drugs on the market, we don't know the true answer to this. We do not know whether using pramlintide for many years will cause more good than harm. It often takes five or ten years of use in many thousands of people before we know the answer to that. What we do know is that when you start taking pramlintide, you may notice that you are less hungry, and so it is easier to eat the right amount of food. You may find that your blood glucose does not rise so fast after a meal and that your blood glucose stays closer to normal for longer after the meal. You may need to reduce your dose of insulin when you start taking pramlintide. Some people lose some weight when they add pramlintide to their diabetes regimen.

What are the problems with pramlintide (Symlin)?

Pramlintide is only useful if you are already taking insulin. It must be given as a separate injection from insulin and should never be mixed with your insulin. The most common side effect is nausea. This is worse in the first few weeks of taking it. I usually advise people to start at a low dose (just 15 mcg injected before any meal containing at least 30 grams of carbohydrate). The dose can be gradually increased over six or eight weeks to a maximum dose of 120 mcg before each meal. Taking pramlintide increases your risk of having hypoglycemia. You will probably need to reduce your insulin dose when you start pramlintide. Exactly how much to reduce by is difficult to predict. You should only use pramlintide if you are seeing a doctor who has experience with using it. No one knows if using pramlintide for many years will cause more good than harm.

Chapter 28

Traveling and Diabetes

- Is it okay to travel if I have diabetes?
- Will customs officials in other countries think I am a drug addict if I am carrying needles and syringes?
- Will they have my kind of insulin or pills or glucose testing supplies in a foreign country?
- Should I take extra supplies with me when I am traveling?
- How do I deal with my insulin shots if I am traveling across different time zones?

Is it okay to travel if I have diabetes?

Absolutely. If you have no other health problems that might make it hard for you to travel, there is no reason why having diabetes should stop you from traveling. Exactly how difficult it will be for you depends on the type of diabetes you have, where you are traveling to, and how long you will be gone.

Here are some general pieces of advice. Take identification with you explaining that you have diabetes. You may want to ask your doctor to supply you with a letter explaining what treatment you take for your diabetes. Check your insurance coverage and have emergency contact phone numbers with you in case you get sick. If you are unsure what the food will be like where you are going, you should take a supply of both simple and complex carbohydrate with you to supplement the food you will be given. You can ask for special meals on your plane flights. Take all of your pills, insulin, syringes, needles, insulin pens, blood glucose testing supplies, and anything else that you need to manage your diabetes with you in your carry-on luggage so that it is with you at all times.

The American Diabetes Association has some very useful and practical tips at http://diabetes.org/advocacy-and-legalresources/discrimination/public_accommodation/travel.jsp. Another way to get that information is to go to the main ADA website (http://diabetes.org) and type the word "travel" in the search engine box.

Will customs officials in other countries think I am a drug addict if I am carrying needles and syringes?

Hopefully not! Within the United States, this is not likely at all. The American Diabetes Association has worked closely with the Transportation Security Administration (TSA), the government agency that is in charge of screening at airports. You should tell them that you have diabetes and that you have all of your supplies with you. You can offer to show these to the screeners at the airport so that it is clear to them that you are not trying to hide anything. It may be helpful to have a letter with you from your doctor and also to have the prescription labels on your pills, insulin, and supplies. If you use tubes of glucose gel to treat hypoglycemia, these should be in containers or tubes less than three ounces.

Will they have my kind of insulin or pills or glucose testing supplies in a foreign country?

That is hard to say. It depends on where you are going. Many countries in the world have sophisticated medical systems and will have a wide variety of drugs and insulin available to treat diabetes. However, I strongly recommend that you take plenty of everything that you will need with you so that you will not have to rely on getting diabetic supplies in a foreign country unless it is a real emergency. If you are going to a country with a warm climate, then you need to make sure that you keep your insulin and blood glucose test equipment cool.

Should I take extra supplies with me when I am traveling?

Definitely. I recommend that you take twice as much of everything that you think you will need. If you are traveling with someone else, it is a good idea to have the other person carry everything you might need and for you to do the same. That way if your luggage gets lost or stolen, you will still have what you need. In addition to your usual diabetes supplies (pills, insulin, blood glucose testing equipment, ketostix, glucose tablets, and snacks), it is a good idea to bring anti-diarrhea and anti-nausea medicine with you, extra fluids, batteries for your blood glucose meter, and a "Sharps" container to dispose of your needles, syringes, and lancets.

How do I deal with my insulin shots if I am traveling across different time zones?

It is difficult to give you specific advice about this, because it depends on what types of insulin you are taking, how big the doses are, how many time zones you are traveling through, and whether you are flying east to west, or west to east. The key thing to do is to check your blood glucose frequently and make adjustments that make sense. You will not get much exercise on the plane, so your blood glucose might be higher than usual. If you are stressed about the journey, this will also push your blood glucose up. Because you will keep your insulin supplies with you, it should be fairly easy to take extra shots of insulin to cover all your extra airplane meals and to bring down your glucose if it gets too high. Remember that airplane flights are air-conditioned, and so you can get very dry. Make sure you drink plenty of water to stay hydrated.

Let me give you an example that I talk to my patients about a lot. If you live on the West Coast of the United States and are traveling to the United Kingdom, you "lose" eight hours on the flight to the UK and "gain" eight hours on the way back. Let's say you take Regular insulin (which lasts up to six or eight hours) and NPH insulin (which lasts about twelve hours or more) twice a day (at about 8:00 a.m. and 8:00 p.m.). It usually works to take your usual doses of Regular and NPH on the morning of your flight to the UK. However, it will only be sixteen hours later until it will be 8:00 a.m. in the UK again! It usually works best to take only Regular insulin (every four to six hours) until you get to the UK. You can then take your next dose of the longer-acting NPH insulin when it is 8:00 a.m. in the UK.

On the way back, it will seem like a really long day. When you take your morning dose of Regular and NPH insulin on the day you leave the UK, it will be thirty-two hours until it will be 8:00 a.m. the next day back on the West Coast of the United States. It usually works well to take your second dose of NPH insulin twelve hours after your first dose of NPH and then take an extra dose of Regular insulin about twelve hours after that. That should tide you over until you get back to the United States and take your next dose of NPH at 8:00 a.m. Pacific standard time. I hope that makes sense. If you are confused about what to do, please talk to your diabetes doctor or nurse about it so that you can work out a plan that makes sense.

Chapter 29 ALTERNATIVE THERAPIES

- What are the best herbal supplements for someone with diabetes?
- How will I know if a new supplement for diabetes is helping me or not?
- Do people with diabetes need to take vitamins?
- Should I take extra vitamin E?
- Does alpha-lipoic acid help diabetic nerve damage?
- Will prescription medicines and over-the-counter drugs work differently if I have diabetes?
- Will chromium or vanadium help lower my blood glucose?
- Can I be sure that supplements contain what it says on the bottle?
- If an herbal preparation contains lots of things, how do I know which ones are most effective?
- Can herbal preparations revive the pancreas and make it start working again?
- Does glucosamine make your blood glucose go up?
- Does cinnamon make your blood glucose go down?
- Are alternative therapies ever harmful?
- Why are people with diabetes told to get flu shots and pneumonia shots?

What are the best herbal supplements for someone with diabetes?

Because diabetes is so common, you will be bombarded by ads from people trying to sell you things to "help you" manage your diabetes. Companies that make herbal supplements and the products that they sell are growing in number. Everything from Chinese cucumber to cinnamon bark is supposed to help you. While some of the claims are based on sensible ideas and research, a lot of the claims are not. A good, reliable source of information is the National Center for Complementary and Alternative Medicine (http://nccam.nih.gov/health/diabetes/).

How will I know if a new supplement for diabetes is helping me or not?

The idea of taking a "natural supplement" is very appealing to many people, especially if they are frustrated because the things they are doing right now for their diabetes are not working well enough. Many of the natural herbal supplements are marketed very effectively and have an appealing and plausible story behind them. If you feel as though something will help and are convinced that it is safe and healthy for you, then you are much more likely to believe that it is doing you good. When people are given placebo (or "dummy") pills as part of a research study, they almost always show improvement in their symptoms. Because of this, it is hard to know if a new herbal supplement is helping you or not. Many of the herbal supplements on the market have not been tested using well-designed, randomized, placebo-controlled, double-blind clinical trials.

Here is an approach that I suggest you try if you are interested in taking a new supplement. Before you start taking it, try to do all the things you are already doing as well as possible (check your blood glucose several times a day, eat a healthy diet, get regular exercise, and take all your medicines as they were prescribed). After three weeks of this, start adding the new supplement while continuing to do everything else as well as you can. After a few more weeks, if you are convinced that your blood glucose levels are now even better than they were before, then by all means continue to take the new supplement. But if you do not notice that anything is improved, there is no need to waste your money on the new supplement.

Do people with diabetes need to take vitamins?

Most people who eat a healthy and balanced diet will get enough minerals and vitamins to keep themselves healthy. You are not any more likely to need vitamins just because you have diabetes. However, if you want to be sure that you are getting enough of all of the vitamins and minerals that you need, it is reasonable to take a "one-a-day" multivitamin that has 100 percent of the recommended daily amount for all of the essential vitamins and minerals. There are several on the market that you can get over the counter and quite cheaply. You will find multivitamins that are marketed as being specially designed for women or specially designed for people with diabetes, but there is no evidence that they are any more beneficial than a regular multivitamin. They are likely to be more expensive, however, because they have been "specially designed."

Should I take extra vitamin E?

Vitamin E has been heavily marketed in the past few years as being one of the "antioxidant vitamins" that you should take in much higher doses than the recommended daily amount. Like most antioxidant supplements, the marketing "pitch" talks about the ability of antioxidants to get rid of "free radicals" in your body. Several large, well-designed, randomized clinical trials have looked at whether adding high doses of vitamin E to your diet will result in fewer heart attacks or other health benefits. The results of all of these studies, so far, show no benefit from taking extra vitamin E.

Does alpha-lipoic acid help diabetic nerve damage?

Some part of diabetic nerve damage may be due to "oxidative stress," and so a potent antioxidant like alpha-lipoic acid may be helpful. In a randomized, placebo-controlled clinical trial, when people with painful diabetic neuropathy were given alpha-lipoic acid, they got improvement in stabbing, burning pain and numbness during five weeks of treatment. Even the lowest dose (600 mg) gave improvement. The higher doses gave no more benefit but caused more side effects (like nausea, vomiting, and a spinning sensation of dizziness). We don't know if alpha-lipoic acid will work for longer periods but it may be worth while trying 600 mg, especially if you have stabbing or burning pain and you do not want to use drugs like tricyclic antidepressants or gabapentin. You should talk to your doctor before you add alpha-lipoic acid to your daily treatment.

Will prescription medicines and over-the-counter drugs work differently if I have diabetes?

Most prescription medicines and over-the-counter drugs will work just as well in someone with diabetes as in anyone else. Over-the-counter cough medicines and syrups that contain a lot of sugar may make your blood glucose go up if you take a lot of it, but there are several brands that use artificial sweeteners. It is possible that some of the drugs that you are taking for your diabetes might interact with other drugs that are prescribed for you, but most pharmacists will check what other things you are taking and double-check with computer databases to see if there might be problems. If your diabetes has caused problems with your heart or liver or kidneys, that could interfere with some other prescription medicines and over-the-counter drugs. It is best to double-check with your own doctor before adding a new medicine.

Will chromium or vanadium help lower my blood glucose?

The idea of using chromium for diabetes is an interesting story. Chromium is an essential trace element. In other words, we all need to have some chromium in our diet in order to metabolize glucose properly. If people become chromium deficient, they can develop diabetes. This can happen to starving children in Third World countries and can also occur in certain parts of the world where there is very little chromium in the diet. In these situations, treating people with supplements of chromium will reverse (or at least improve) their diabetes. This has been shown in randomized, controlled clinical trials in China, for example. However, it is extremely unlikely that a healthy, middle-class American or European person is deficient in chromium. Research trials in this country have not shown that adding chromium to the diet of most American patients with type 2 diabetes improves anything very much at all.

Vanadium is another heavy metal that can affect your glucose level by altering metabolism inside your cells. It is unlikely that you have vanadium deficiency or that you will benefit from adding vanadium to your diet, but you can try it and see if you think it helps.

Can I be sure that supplements contain what it says on the bottle?

No. That is one of the biggest problems with herbal supplements: they are not regulated by a government agency like the Federal Drug Administration, and often there is no quality control to make sure that every batch of supplement that is packaged up and sold contains the same amount of "active ingredient" as the last batch. In a recent study published in the *New England Journal of Medicine,* researchers tested several different brands of supplement (like ginseng) and found that the actual amounts in the supplement could vary by two to ten times what was stated on the bottle. Sometimes there was much less active ingredient than the bottle stated, and at other times there was more. In at least one or two cases, they found that the only reason the "natural supplement" lowered blood glucose levels was because the unscrupulous manufacturers had added an active blood glucose lowering drug (glyburide) to the "natural supplement."

I don't want you to think that all of the companies who manufacture natural supplements are dangerous or untrustworthy. Many of them are very careful about how they prepare their supplements and are very genuine in believing that their product will be good for you. You should be cautious and get your supplements from a source that you think is reliable.

If an herbal preparation contains lots of things, how do I know which ones are most effective?

This can be really difficult. Many herbal supplements contain a very long list of "ingredients," and there is no way to test them one by one. The best advice I can give is to try to buy from a source that you think is reputable and test your blood glucose before, during, and after you give yourself a one-month trial of the new herbal preparation. If you are convinced that you feel better, and if you can show that your blood glucose levels have improved, then it might be worth continuing to take the herbal preparation, even if you are not sure what particular ingredients are being most effective.

Can herbal preparations revive the pancreas and make it start working again?

No, they can't, and anyone who claims such a thing is a crook. In my thirty years of being a diabetes doctor, I can remember two times when young patients of mine with type 1 diabetes were deceived by a company that claimed their supplement could cure their diabetes and make their pancreas start working again. On both occasions, these young people stopped taking their insulin shots, threw away their syringes and needles, and started taking the new natural herbal supplements instead. In less than forty-eight hours, they were feeling terrible and had to be admitted to hospital with really high blood glucose levels. One of them passed out into a coma due to diabetic ketoacidosis. Both of them recovered when they were given an incredible natural supplement that their bodies were lacking…insulin.

Does glucosamine make your blood glucose go up?

Glucosamine is a molecule that is used to make cartilage and connective tissue in your body. It can be used to help with joint and muscle aches and pains. We do not know if it works because it repairs cartilage or connective tissue or not. It also has mild anti-inflammatory effects. It can be used along with chondroitin and has been shown in some clinical trials to improve joint pain, especially in people with severe osteoarthritis and cartilage loss. Animal studies have shown that glucosamine may increase insulin resistance, and so it is possible that your blood glucose may go up while you are taking it. This is not usually a major problem.

Several of my patients who have diabetes did not notice any change in their blood glucose levels after starting glucosamine. I suggest that if you plan to start taking glucosamine, you check your blood glucose levels regularly before you start taking it, and then see if you can tell any difference in the first week or two of starting to take glucosamine. If you do, you should talk to your doctor about it. It may be possible to change the dose of your diabetes pills or insulin in order to keep taking the glucosamine without your blood glucose going up.

Does cinnamon make your blood glucose go down?

Some small research studies (including one from Pakistan in 2003) have suggested that taking cinnamon three times a day after meals might help lower your blood glucose. There is hot debate about which type of cinnamon is most effective and how much you need to take. About a teaspoon (or 5 grams) of the spicy, ground-up tree bark seems to be a popular choice. As with many other alternative therapies, the scientific evidence for this is a bit weak, but it probably won't hurt you to try adding some cinnamon to your diet (after making sure you are doing everything else as well as you can before you add the cinnamon). The problem is that cinnamon is not very pleasant to take unless it is mixed up with sugar and is served on apple pie or in a cinnamon roll!

Are alternative therapies ever harmful?

Yes, they can be, although it is rare. Most companies who make natural supplements are very genuine and make supplements that are at least harmless and might even do you some good. But if the company has spiked its "natural supplement" with a drug like glyburide to make sure that your blood glucose goes down, and if you have an allergy to sulfa-drugs, then you could become very ill if you took it. And if a company convinced you to stop taking all of your diabetes pills or insulin shots, the results could be extremely harmful.

Why are people with diabetes told to get flu shots and pneumonia shots?

Most people with diabetes are not any more likely to get the flu or pneumonia than people who do not have diabetes. However, if you have diabetes and you do get the flu or pneumonia, then it can be more serious for you. These are serious infections. They can cause a lot of insulin resistance. You feel so awful (with aches, pains, high fever, and nausea) that you may not feel like eating or drinking enough fluids. All of this can push your blood glucose up to dangerous levels and can cause diabetic ketoacidosis, a very serious condition that often needs to be treated in hospital. Because of that, it is a good idea for anyone with diabetes to get flu and pneumonia shots.

Influenza is a virus that changes slightly every year, and so you need to get a flu shot every year. The pneumonia shot protects you against one particular bacterium that can cause pneumonia (called pneumococcal pneumonia). A single pneumonia shot protects you for at least five years and possibly longer. Although getting flu and pneumonia shots will protect you against influenza virus and pneumococcal bacteria, there are other viruses and bacteria that can infect your lungs, so it is important to take other precautions to protect yourself (like washing your hands regularly and keeping your diabetes well controlled).

Part Four: Staying Positive

Chapter 30

Making a Good Plan

- Is having diabetes my fault?
- Is it normal to get frustrated with my diabetes?
- How can I remember all of the things I am supposed to do?
- What are the most important things to focus on with my diabetes?
- How can I get the most out of my relationship with my health care team?
- How often should I get a physical?
- How often should I get laboratory tests?
- How often should I see my diabetes doctor?
- How can I tell if new treatments that I hear about in the media would be good ones for me?

Is having diabetes my fault?

Absolutely not. Nobody gets diabetes just because they ate the wrong things or let their weight creep up or didn't exercise enough. You only get diabetes if you have a problem with your pancreas or have inherited the genes for type 1 or type 2 diabetes from your parents. It is not going to help you or anyone else if you spend time blaming yourself. It isn't a good idea to blame your parents, either! It is just one of those things.

If you have diabetes, the quicker you accept it, the quicker you can focus your energy and attention on how to deal with it well. That means understanding what type of diabetes you have and what things you can do to improve your future health. You need to be able to incorporate diabetes into your everyday life and do what you can to live a long and healthy life with diabetes. Filling your head with guilt or blame is not a good use of your time and energy. There are lots of things that you can do to manage your diabetes well. Focus your energy on those.

Is it normal to get frustrated with my diabetes?

Definitely. Living with diabetes every day can really drive you nuts. People who don't have diabetes can't really understand what a drag it is to have to think about what you eat, how often you have to check your blood glucose, when to take your pills or give yourself insulin. There is a lot of stuff to remember to do. What is even more frustrating is that even when you do all of those things perfectly, your blood glucose readings will still sometimes make no sense to you.

I often get asked to see someone with diabetes because their doctor has said, "Mrs. Hernandez is noncompliant! She has stopped measuring her blood glucose every morning the way I told her to. See if you can fix her." A note like that always tells me much more about the doctor than the patient. Often when I sit down with Mrs.

Hernandez and ask her what is bothering her about her diabetes she will say, "Dr. McCulloch, I do everything like I'm supposed to. I eat all the right things, do my exercise, take my medicines, and go to bed with a pretty good blood glucose level—but every morning when I wake up, my blood glucose is really high again. There is nothing I can do that helps, so I just stopped testing."

To me, the problem is not that Mrs. Hernandez is being "bad" or "noncompliant" because she is not doing what her doctor told her to. The problem is that her doctor is not helping her to fix the problem. Mrs. Hernandez has every right to be frustrated. It doesn't make any sense at all to keep pricking your finger to put a drop of blood onto expensive blood glucose strips if the results frustrate you and you have no way to improve the situation. What Mrs. Hernandez needs is to switch to a doctor who can help her to understand why her glucose readings are too high and then help her to fix the problem. Then she will feel less frustrated.

How can I remember all of the things I am supposed to do?

It is hard to remember everything, especially if you are on a lot of medications, all for different things, and if you see a lot of different doctors and other health care professionals for different conditions. You can write things down in a diary or on the calendar. You can keep a list of all your medications, when to take them, and what they are for. You can write down your blood glucose readings in a book and mark how much carbohydrate you eat or when you exercise or how much insulin you take. There are a lot of different approaches that work for different people.

One thing that might help you is to develop a summary of everything that you are supposed to do and to write down what matters to you, what your goals are, and who you should call for different things. This is sometimes called a "Care Plan" or a "Shared Care Plan," since it is something that you might want to share with your family or with other doctors who are seeing you for the first time. You might find it helpful to look at examples of how other people go about this. You will get a lot of useful information at www.sharedcareplan.org.

What are the most important things to focus on with my diabetes?

I think that a better question to ask yourself is, "What do I love to do?" or "What are my personal goals for the next few months or years?" or "What do I most want to do in my life that I haven't been able to?" Then you can ask yourself, "What is it about my diabetes that is preventing me from doing those things?" Instead of feeling that diabetes is dominating your life, you can try to think how best to fit diabetes into the rest of your life.

The most important thing to focus on first is feeling as well as you can from day to day. Are you depressed or frustrated with your diabetes? Can you keep your blood glucose from being so high that you are thirsty and tired all the time and from being so low that you are sweaty, shaky, and unable to think straight? Can you remember to take your pills or your insulin shots and check your blood glucose often enough that it is helpful to you?

If you are coping with diabetes from day to day, the next question to ask is, "What are all the things that I can do to stay as healthy as possible both now and in the future?" For most adults with diabetes, the biggest risk to your health is from heart disease, so doing what you can to lower your risk of heart disease is a really important thing to focus on. I went over this in detail in other parts of the book. You should quit smoking, eat a healthy diet, get some exercise, try to do something fun to keep your stress level down. You should get your blood pressure, cholesterol, and HbA1c checked. You should talk to your doctor about whether you should be taking aspirin, a statin drug, and an ACE-inhibitor. You should ask if you need to get your eyes, feet, and kidneys checked every year. In truth, one of the most important things for you to focus on is having a good relationship with your health care team.

How can I get the most out of my relationship with my health care team?

Finding someone whom you connect with and who "gets" who you are and what matters to you is really important. Just like in other important relationships in your life, there are some indefinable qualities about this. You can sometimes just "tell" if this doctor or nurse is someone you can relate to or not.

How do you like to communicate: by phone, by email, in writing, in person? What options does your health care team offer you for communication? Clear communication is a key thing to building a good relationship. Do you need to come in for this visit, or could you get your questions answered by phone or email? If you are coming in for a visit, what is the purpose, and how long will you have with your health care team? If you have a lot of questions, it is good to write them down in case you forget when you are with your health care team. Do you really have a team? Does your doctor work with a nurse or dietitian or pharmacist who understands about diabetes and is part of the team? If so, which is the best person to ask about different concerns you have?

I love using email with my patients, not as a replacement for face-to-face visits but as a way to enhance them. I encourage my patients to email me or write to me before we meet so that I know what questions and concerns they have. If the list is really long, I can make sure I have enough time, or I will suggest a longer appointment or that we only talk about some of them at this visit and make another appointment to go over the rest.

It is important for you to be able to see your health care team when you have a particular problem or concern. But even if you feel fine, I think it is a good idea to have at least one visit a year to go over the "big picture." This is a good time to update your Care Plan, if you have one. You can go over your life goals or the targets for your HbA1c, blood pressure, cholesterol, for example. You can make sure that you are up to date with your eye exams and foot exams. It gives you an opportunity to ask about any new drugs or tests that you have heard of.

Hopefully your health care team will be enthusiastic about helping you with all of these things and might even keep track of when you are coming due for eye exams and other screening tests. If not, then you might be better looking for a new doctor and health care team that you can work better with.

How often should I get a physical?

This is a tricky thing to answer, because it depends so much on how healthy you are. Some people like the reassurance of getting an "annual physical," as if this gives you some kind of guarantee that you are healthy, like when you take your car in for a checkup every five thousand miles. But in truth, when you take your car in they don't check everything. They check some specific things like your oil and fluid levels, the wear and tear on your tires, and how well your brakes work, for example. The same is true for a "physical." It may make you feel better to have a doctor listen to your heart and lungs or press on your belly, but unless you have specific symptoms, doing those things doesn't always do much to keep you healthy.

If you have diabetes and are feeling well, it still makes sense to have your feet examined at least once a year to see that the sensation on your feet is normal, that the shape of your feet is normal, and that the circulation is good. It makes sense to have an eye exam by a trained optometrist or ophthalmologist every year or two to make sure that your eyes are healthy. Screening your eyes and feet make sense, because it is possible for them to get damaged without you knowing about it. If problems are detected earlier, the treatments to keep you healthy are much easier than if you wait until you have an ulcer on your foot or you notice you can't see as well as you used to. Checking your blood pressure at least once a year also makes sense for the same reason. Your blood pressure might be too high, but you wouldn't know about it unless you check it yourself with a blood pressure machine or come in and get your blood pressure checked as part of a physical. But apart from checking those specific things, I am not sure that a physical exam is very helpful unless you have new symptoms or concerns.

How often should I get laboratory tests?

It depends on how old you are, what other medical conditions you have, and what treatment you are on. You should know what your HbA1c level is, when it was last checked, and what target you are trying to reach. If you are above this target, then your HbA1c should be checked every three months, and you should be making changes to how you manage your diabetes until you get to your target. If you are already at your HbA1c target, it is still a good idea to have your HbA1c checked once or twice a year to make sure it stays there. If your body gradually makes less insulin, or if you become more stressed or resistant to insulin, then your HbA1c might drift up. You will get quite a good idea how your overall blood glucose is doing by doing your own blood glucose tests, but keeping track of your HbA1c is also a good idea.

You should probably get a urine test for microalbuminuria once a year to check how well your kidneys are doing. A blood test for creatinine is another helpful kidney test to check on. It is good to know what your LDL cholesterol, HDL cholesterol, and triglycerides are. You may not need to get these done every year. It depends on your age and whether you are on treatment to keep them in a normal range. It is easier to remember to get things checked once a year; but in truth, some things don't need to be checked that often, and other things need to be checked more often than once a year.

Depending on what drugs you are on, it might be good to get your potassium checked or a test to see how well your liver is doing. This test is sometimes called a liver function test, or LFT. The laboratory measures how much of the enzyme alanine aminotransferase (ALT) is in your blood. If your liver is inflamed or irritated, then it releases more ALT into your blood. This can sometimes be due to a drug that you are taking, but the ALT can also be higher than normal if your blood glucose level is too high.

How often should I see my diabetes doctor?

It depends on how complicated your diabetes treatment is, how confident you are about what you are doing, and how much support you feel that you need or want. You certainly ought to be seen at least once a year for a planned visit. Even if you have already got the eye, foot, and blood pressure checks and the laboratory tests that I mentioned, it is still a good thing to go over your goals and targets with your doctor at least once a year. If you are having frustrations or are making changes to your treatment, then you may need to be seen more often than once a year. Some doctors (and books) recommend that you should be seen every three months if you have diabetes, but I don't think that is always true. How often you are seen should depend on what you want to get out of the visit.

How can I tell if new treatments that I hear about in the media would be good ones for me?

It is getting more and more common for pharmaceutical companies to advertise directly to consumers. The new drug always sounds great, of course. How can you tell if it really would be good for you? One approach is to use reputable sources for getting your information. Websites like the American Diabetes Association are likely to be less biased than a pharmaceutical company's own website, for example. It also helps to look at the information being presented very carefully. Don't be taken in. Don't accept things at face value.

Let me give you some practice. Let's say a pharmaceutical company called PharmDrug, Inc., does a marketing splash for their new "wonder drug" called Fixitol. Everywhere you go, you see ads for Fixitol: "FIXITOL fixes everything in your life! A recent randomized, double-blind, placebo-controlled clinical trial showed that taking FIXITOL improved everything by a dramatic 300 percent compared to placebo! Only 10 percent of patients had significant side effects. Ask your doctor about FIXITOL!" Sounds too good to be true, right? Well, you know what they say, "If something seems too good to be true…it probably is!"

Let me explain what some of these technical words actually mean and then show you how, without actually lying, PharmDrug, Inc. could be misleading you. If a trial is "randomized," this means that people who take part are picked at random to either get the new treatment (in our example they would be given the new drug Fixitol) or not. If the clinical trial uses a "placebo," this means that the people who don't get Fixitol will get a pill that looks identical to Fixitol but has no active ingredients in it (a placebo is sometimes called a "dummy pill" or "sugar pill"). When a trial is "double-blind," this means that nobody knows who is taking the real Fixitol and who is taking the dummy pill. The participants don't know and neither do the doctors and nurses looking after them. This is really important, since you are more likely to feel better if you think you are taking the real drug, and the doctors and nurses are likely to treat you differently if they know that you are on the real drug.

A randomized, double-blind, placebo-controlled clinical trial is the best way to test a new drug. It is the "gold standard." But even if the clinical trial used this approach, it is still possible for PharmDrug, Inc., to mislead you by the way they report the results. Let's say that two thousand people participated. One thousand of them took Fixitol, and one thousand took the placebo pills. One person in the placebo group said that "everything was better" at the end of the trial, and three people in the Fixitol group said that "everything was better." It is technically correct to say that this is a threefold difference (or a 300 percent improvement) between Fixitol and the placebo. But only four people out of the two thousand who participated in the clinical trial actually got any benefit at all. So only 0.3 percent of people taking Fixitol got any benefit, and the other 99.7 percent didn't. Doctors would need to put five hundred people on Fixitol in order to be sure that one of them would get any benefit.

And what about those side effects? First of all what do they mean by "significant" side effects? They may make light of symptoms that you would find unpleasant. And to say that "only" 10 percent of participants got side effects means that one hundred people who took Fixitol felt worse on it. So the real results of this well-designed clinical trial are that for every five hundred people who start on Fixitol, fifty will get side effects that make them feel worse, and only one will get better. When you put it like that, Fixitol doesn't seem like such a great drug to take, does it?

If you want more information from a reliable source check out http://clinicaltrials.gov/info/resources. If you are interested in understanding more details about the statistics used by pharmaceutical companies, you can find books as simple as *Statistics for Dummies* all the way to college-level textbooks.

Chapter 31

Getting Support

- How much should my family and friends know about diabetes?
- Should I tell my coworkers about my diabetes?
- What should I do when I get frustrated and depressed about my diabetes?
- How can I tell if I am really depressed or not?
- Does diabetes affect your sex drive?
- What are the most reliable sources of information on diabetes?

How much should my family and friends know about diabetes?

The best answer is, "As much as you want them to know and as much as you think they can cope with and understand in order to be helpful to you." You need to use your own judgment. A distant relative whom you are not close to doesn't need to know much of anything, but for people you sleep with or live close to, it can be very helpful to you if they understand something about what it is like for you having diabetes. You should all be eating the same, healthy diet, for example. If you take pills or insulin that are likely to push your blood glucose down below normal from time to time, then your close family ought to know how to tell that your blood glucose is too low and what they can do to help you bring your blood glucose up. If there is a chance you could pass out unconscious from hypoglycemia during the night, then it might be helpful to have a close family member know how to give you an injection of glucagon to bring you out of it. If you have younger children who might be scared by this or would be too young to give you an injection, you could still ask them to call 9–1-1 or a neighbor or friend.

Should I tell my coworkers about my diabetes?

Again, you need to decide how much it matters. If you have to take time off from work to go to a lot of doctors' appointments, you might want to tell your boss and your coworkers so that they won't think you are just being lazy! If you work with dangerous equipment and could put other people in danger if you became confused or drowsy because of a low blood glucose, it would be a good idea to tell them so that they can help you. It is a good idea to wear identification (in your wallet or as a MedicAlert bracelet) telling a stranger that you have diabetes, so that if you are in an accident, people will know.

It really depends on the situation you are in. Ask yourself, "What are the advantages to other people knowing that I have diabetes? How bad would it be for me if I passed out and nobody knew I had diabetes? How likely is that? Will my boss and coworkers treat me differently if they know I have diabetes?"

What should I do when I get frustrated and depressed about my diabetes?

It is completely normal to get frustrated and depressed about having diabetes. Diabetes puts restrictions and burdens on you that interfere with your everyday life. There are likely to be days when you are just sick of it and want to forget about it completely and pretend you don't have diabetes. Maybe that's how you feel most days.

Many books have been written on this topic. Here are two that many of my patients have found to be helpful: *Psyching Out Diabetes: A Positive Approach to Your Negative Emotions* by Richard R. Rubin and *Diabetes Burnout: What to Do When You Can't Take It Anymore* by William H. Polonsky. Dick Rubin and Bill Polonsky are both clinical psychologists and certified diabetes educators. They are also incredibly warm and down-to-earth human beings who have spent years working with people with diabetes and helping them overcome their frustrations. You will find many practical tips and approaches in these books.

There are two aspects of your frustration that you should think about. The first thing to do is find one or more people with whom you can share your frustration. Do you know some other people who have diabetes? Does your local clinic or hospital offer support groups? You will be amazed at how much better you feel when you hear other people describing some of the same things that have frustrated you. You may be surprised at how much you have figured out that you didn't realize. You may find yourself offering suggestions to help other people with diabetes and hearing new things to try from them.

This brings me to the second thing to focus on when you feel frustrated. Try to be very specific about what things are frustrating you. Make a list. How many things on that list are really due to your diabetes, and how many are caused by other things in your life? Try to think up possible solutions for some of them. If the problem is that you don't understand why a certain thing is happening, try to find out. The answers in this book are an attempt to explain some common frustrations that you may have. And if you have figured out why something is frustrating you about your diabetes, see if you can come up with some new ideas for things that you could do differently that might help.

A very popular and useful support group that offers structured and practical advice is called "Living Well with Chronic Illness." These groups were developed by Dr. Kate Lorig and her colleagues at Stanford University and are available in more than twenty-seven states in the United States. They provide a wonderful opportunity to share ideas with other people who are dealing with some of the same frustrations as you. Ask at your local clinic or hospital if these support groups are available near you.

How can I tell if I am really depressed or not?

Sometimes it can be really hard to tell. You may just be feeling hopeless and frustrated and feel that you have no way out of your situation. Here are some things to ask yourself. Are you having trouble falling asleep? Do you feel as if you have no energy, you can't concentrate, and you are tired all the time? Are you losing interest in doing things that used to give you pleasure? Have you no interest in food? Are you overeating? Are you feeling bad about yourself and as though you have let yourself and other people down?

Although none of these things by itself means you are depressed, if you answered "yes" to more than one of them, you should talk to your doctor so that he or she can do a more complete evaluation. Having depression is a real illness, just like getting influenza or pneumonia. It is not your fault. It is nothing to be ashamed about or blame yourself for. It can be treated. In fact, if it is not treated, it will be hard for you to be successful or happy in any aspect of your life. If you think you may be depressed, please ask for help as soon as possible.

Does diabetes affect your sex drive?

Yes, it can. People usually feel most romantic and interested in sex when they are relaxed and can be spontaneous. It is hard to feel like that if you are embarrassed that you have lumps and bruises from where you give your insulin shots or if you are worried about your blood glucose dropping too low. It is not very romantic to tell your partner to stop in the middle of lovemaking so that you can check your blood glucose. If your diabetes is out of control and you feel exhausted, stressed, and thirsty, this will affect your sex drive. If you have a yeast infection and need to go to the bathroom a lot, this can interfere with sex. Whether you have diabetes or not the most important thing to do to help your sex drive is to have good communication with your partner. There is no reason you can't have as healthy and enjoyable a sex life as anyone without diabetes. Just like with other aspects of life, having diabetes means there are more things for you to think about and adjust, but with a loving partner and a good attitude, your sex drive should be as good as anyone else's. If it is not, you should talk to your doctor about it.

What are the most reliable sources of information on diabetes?

I have mentioned several sources throughout this book that will give you reliable information. For most of these I have given websites rather than phone numbers. Information is likely to be more reliable and less biased if it is from a federal, state, or local government site or from a charitable organization (like the American Diabetes Association or the Juvenile Diabetes Research Foundation), rather than from a commercial company that makes money from selling diabetes drugs and supplies. If you do not have access to the internet, then I suggest you contact your local health department and ask for diabetes information. Here is a list of the websites that I have mentioned throughout the book:

- The American Diabetes Association www.diabetes.org
- The Juvenile Diabetes Research Foundation www.jdrf.org
- Continuous glucose monitoring systems: www.dexcom.com or www.medtronic.com or www.glucowatch.com
- Quitting smoking: www.freeclear.com
- Emergency identification: www.medicalert.com
- Portion size: www.platemethod.com
- Carbohydrate counting: www.calorieking.com
- Walking and pedometers: www.walkamerica.org or www.americaonthemove.org or www.10kaday.com or www. shapeup.org
- Insulin pumps: www.diabetes.org/type-1-diabetes/ insulin-pumps.jsp
- Alternate and complementary therapies: nccam.nih.gov/health/diabetes/
- Shared Care Plans: www.sharedcareplan.org
- Research and clinical trials: www.clinicaltrials.gov/info/ resources

Let me give you one last resource that you might find helpful. I have tried to answer all the common questions that I get about diabetes in this book. I asked a few dozen people I know who have diabetes themselves or who work with people who have diabetes. Their questions have also been included in the book. But it may be that you still have questions that did not appear in the book and that you would like to have answered. Maybe you have follow-up questions. I have set up a weblog to accompany this book. If you have more questions, I invite you to write to me at www.morediabetesanswers.com. I will do my best to read your questions and post answers that anyone can look at. And if we end up doing a second edition of *The Diabetes Answer Book,* then I will include the best of these new questions in that book.

Glossary

A1c (or glycosylated hemoglobin or hemoglobin A1c or HbA1c)—a blood test that measures the average blood glucose level over the previous eight to twelve weeks

A-chain—one of the two chemical chains that make up the insulin molecule

Acanthosis nigricans—a skin condition that is sometimes found in people who have insulin resistance

Acarbose—a drug that slows down the absorption of complex carbohydrates from your guts

ACE-inhibitor—a drug class that helps to lower blood pressure, protect the kidneys, and reduce the risk of heart disease

ACE receptor blocker—a drug class that has similar effects to an ACE-inhibitor but with fewer side effects such as cough

Actos—a trade name for pioglitazone, a drug used to treat insulin resistance

Alanine aminotransferase (ALT)—an enzyme that is made in the liver

Alpha-lipoic acid—a naturally-occurring chemical that is sold as a supplement to help a variety of conditions

Alprostadil—a drug that is used to help men with erectile dysfunction

Amitriptyline—a drug that is used to treat depression and the pain from damaged nerves

Amylase—an enzyme made in the pancreas to help digest food

Amyloid—a chemical substance that builds up inside the insulin-producing cells of the pancreas in people who have type 2 diabetes

Apidra—a trade name for glulisine, a fast-acting insulin analog

Aspart—a fast-acting insulin analog

Atorvastatin—a drug used to treat high cholesterol

Atkins diet—a diet that was promoted by Dr. Robert C. Atkins, containing lots of fat and protein and very little carbohydrate

Avandia—a trade name for rosiglitazone, a drug to treat insulin resistance

B-chain—one of the two chemical chains that make up the insulin molecule

Basal insulin—the low and steady amount of insulin that should be present during sleep and between meals

Beta blocker—a drug class that slows the heart rate and lowers blood pressure

Biguanide—a drug class used to treat insulin resistance

Body mass index (BMI)—a way to describe if someone's weight is appropriate for his or her height

Bolus (insulin spike)—the sharp rise in insulin that should occur during meals

Brittle diabetes—diabetes that is very hard to control because of large unpredictable swings from high to low blood glucose levels

Byetta—a trade name for exenatide, a drug used to treat type 2 diabetes

C-peptide—the chemical molecule that connects to the two chains of the insulin molecule to form proinsulin

Candesartan—an ACE receptor blocker drug used to lower blood pressure, protect the kidneys, and reduce the risk of heart disease

Capsaicin—a drug used to treat the pain from damaged nerves

Carb counting—a technique to adjust diabetes treatment by estimating how much carbohydrate you are about to eat

Carbamazepine—a drug used to treat seizure disorders and the pain from damaged nerves

Carborundum stone—a flat stone used to sharpen metal knives and needles

Care plan (or Shared Care Plan)—a written description of all the information about your medical treatment that you want to share with your family, friends, and health-care team

Carpal tunnel syndrome—a medical condition where nerve damage at the wrist can cause pain and weakness in the hand and arm

Captopril—an ACE-inhibitor drug used to lower blood pressure, protect the kidneys, and reduce the risk of heart disease

Chantix—a trade name for varenicline, a drug used to treat tobacco addiction

Charcot foot—a medical condition where painless bone fracture and deformity is the result of nerve damage

Chlorpropamide—a sulfonylurea drug used to increase insulin production

Cholestyramine—a drug used to treat high cholesterol

Chondroitin—a chemical found in cartilage and sold as a natural supplement to treat joint pain

Chromium—a chemical sold as a natural supplement to lower blood glucose levels

Cialis—the trade name for tadalafil, a drug used to treat erectile dysfunction

Clinitest—a tablet that is used to estimate the amount of glucose in someone's urine

Continuous glucose monitor—a device that measures the glucose level in someone's body every few minutes without having to prick the finger every time

Dawn phenomenon—the rise in certain hormones in your body in the few hours before you wake up

Desipramine—a drug that is used to treat depression and the pain from damaged nerves

Detemir—a long-acting insulin analog

Dexfenfluramine—a drug used to curb appetite

DiaBeta—a trade name for glyburide, a drug used to increase insulin production

Diabetes insipidus—a medical condition in which the person produces large amounts of very dilute and tasteless urine

Diabetes mellitus—a medical condition in which the person produces large amounts of very sweet urine

Diabetes Prevention Program (DPP)—an important medical research study to prevent or delay the onset of type 2 diabetes

Diabetic ketoacidosis—a serious medical condition caused by having too little insulin

Diabinese—a trade name for chlorpropamide, a drug used to increase insulin production

Dietitian—a person with special training to give advice about healthy eating

Dipeptidyl peptidase number 4 (DPP-IV)—an enzyme that inactivates the hormone glucagon-like polypeptide number 1 (GLP-1)

Duloxetine—a drug used to treat the pain from damaged nerves

Enalapril—an ACE-inhibitor drug, used to lower blood pressure, protect the kidneys, and reduce the risk of heart disease

Enteric-coated tablets—drugs that are coated with chemicals that allow the drug to pass through the stomach into the intestines without irritating the lining of the stomach

Erythromycin—an antibiotic that can also be used to speed up stomach emptying

Essential trace element—a simple chemical substance that is usually found in food and is essential for your health

Exenatide—a long-acting analog of glucagon-like polypeptide number 1 (GLP-1)

Exubera—a trade name for one form of powdered inhaled insulin

Ezitimibe—a drug used to treat high cholesterol

Fenfluramine—a drug used to curb appetite

Fenofibrate—a drug used to treat high triglycerides

Fen-phen—a combination of fenfluramine and phentermine, two drugs used to curb appetite

Finger stick blood test—pricking your finger and using a test strip to measure the glucose level in a drop of blood

Fortamet—a trade name for metformin, a drug used to treat insulin resistance

Gabapentin—a drug used to treat the pain from damaged nerves

Gastric emptying studies—a medical procedure to measure how quickly the food you eat leaves your stomach

Gastroparesis—a medical condition where nerve damage causes the stomach to empty more slowly than it should

Gemfibrozil—a drug used to treat high triglycerides

Gestational diabetes—diabetes that comes on during pregnancy and goes away afterwards

Ghrelin—a hormone made in the stomach that affects appetite

Glargine—a long-acting insulin analog

Glibenclamide—another word for glyburide, a drug used to increase insulin production

Glimiperide—a sulfonylurea drug used to increase insulin production

Glipizide—a sulfonylurea drug used to increase insulin production

Glitazone—a class of drug used to treat insulin resistance

Glucagon—a hormone made in the pancreas that counteracts some of the effects of insulin and so raises blood glucose levels

Glucagon-like polypeptide number 1 (GLP-1)—a hormone made in the guts that affects blood glucose levels

Glucophage, Glucophage XL—trade names for metformin, a drug used to treat insulin resistance

Glulisine—a fast-acting insulin analog

Glumetza—a trade name for metformin, a drug used to treat insulin resistance

Glyburide—a sulfonylurea drug used to increase insulin production

Glycemic index—a way to describe how quickly blood glucose rises after eating carbohydrate foods

Glycogen—a large molecule of complex carbohydrate used by your body to store glucose in the liver and in muscles

Glycosylated hemoglobin (hemoglobin A1c or HbA1c or A1c)—a blood test that measures the average blood glucose level over the previous eight to twelve weeks

Glynase—a trade name for glyburide, a sulfonylurea drug used to increase insulin production

Glyset—a trade name for miglitol, a drug that slows down the absorption of complex carbohydrates from your guts

HDL cholesterol—high density lipoprotein cholesterol, sometimes called the "good" cholesterol because it reduces your risk of getting blocked arteries

Hemochromatosis—a medical condition where too much iron gets deposited in some of the organs of your body (including the liver and the pancreas) which can lead to diabetes

Hemodialysis—a medical procedure to filter impurities out of the blood of someone whose kidneys are failing

High density lipoproteins (HDL)—a form of cholesterol that is "good" because it reduces your risk of getting blocked arteries

High-fiber carbohydrate—a form of complex carbohydrate containing soluble fiber which slows down the rise of blood glucose after meals

Humalog—a trade name for lispro, a fast-acting insulin analog

Human Leukocyte Antigen (HLA)—protein markers on the surface of human cells that allow them to be recognized by the immune system

Hyperglycemia—high blood glucose level

Hypoglycemia—low blood glucose level

Idaho Plate Method—a simple tool to help control portion size and promote healthy eating habits

Insulin—a hormone made in the pancreas that helps control the glucose levels in your body

Insulin-making (or insulin-producing) cells—specialized cells in the pancreas where insulin is made, stored, and pushed into your blood

Insulin zinc suspension—a long-acting preparation of insulin for injecting under the skin

Islet cell antibody (ICA)—protein molecules made by your immune system when your body treats the insulin-producing cells in your pancreas as if they were a foreign substance

Islets of Langerhans—groups of specialized cells that are scattered throughout the pancreas and make insulin and other hormones

Isomaltase—an enzyme in your guts that breaks complex carbohydrate into smaller pieces

Januvia—a trade name for sitagliptin, a drug used to lower blood glucose levels

Juvenile diabetes—an old-fashioned term for type 1 diabetes, a type of diabetes that is more common in younger people, caused by the person's own immune system destroying the cells that make insulin

Ketone—a chemical substance produced in your body when you break down fat

Ketostix—test sticks that can be used to detect ketones in your urine

LDL cholesterol—low density lipoprotein cholesterol, sometimes called the "bad" cholesterol

Lantus—a trade name for glargine, a long-acting insulin analog

Levemir—a trade name for detemir, a long-acting insulin analog

Levitra—a trade name for vardenafil, a drug used to treat erectile dysfunction

Lipitor—a trade name for atorvastatin, a drug used to treat high cholesterol

Lipoatrophy—a medical condition where some of the fat cells under the skin shrink in response to repeated insulin injections

Lipohypertrophy—a medical condition where some of the fat cells under the skin swell up in response to repeated insulin injections

Lisinopril—an ACE-inhibitor drug used to lower blood pressure, protect the kidneys, and reduce the risk of heart disease

Lispro—a fast-acting insulin analog

Liver function test (LFT)—a blood test that tells how well your liver is working

Losartan—an ACE receptor blocker drug used to lower blood pressure, protect the kidneys, and reduce the risk of heart disease

Lovastatin—a drug used to treat high cholesterol

Low carb diet—a diet high in protein and fat, but low in carbohydrate

Low density lipoprotein—a form of cholesterol that is "bad" because it increases your risk of getting blocked arteries

Lyrica—a trade name for pregabalin, a drug used to treat the pain from damaged nerves

Maltase—an enzyme in your guts that breaks complex carbohydrate into smaller pieces

Maturity-onset diabetes—an old-fashioned term for type 2 diabetes, a type of diabetes that is more common in older people, caused by the progressive loss of insulin production and increased resistance to insulin

Maturity-onset diabetes of the young (MODY)—an uncommon genetic condition where type 2 diabetes can occur in several family members during childhood

Medicalert bracelet—a bracelet telling others that you have significant medical conditions such as diabetes

Meglitinides—a class of drugs used to increase insulin production

Metformin—a drug used to treat insulin resistance

Metoclopramide—a drug used to treat nausea and gastroparesis

Mevacor—a trade name for lovastatin, a drug used to treat high cholesterol

Microalbuminuria—small amounts of protein in the urine

Micronase—a trade name for glyburide, a drug used to increase insulin production

Miglitol—a drug that slows down the absorption of complex carbohydrate from your guts

Morbid obesity—severe obesity (usually defined as a BMI over 40)

Nateglinide—a drug used to increase insulin production

Net carbs—a nonsensical term which subtracts the grams of fiber from the total amount of carbohydrate that a food contains

Neurontin—a trade name for gabapentin, a drug used to treat pain from nerve damage

Nicotinic acid—a vitamin which, when taken in large amounts, is used to treat high cholesterol

Nortriptyline—a drug used to treat the pain from nerve damage

Novolog—a trade name for aspart, a fast-acting insulin analog

Nutrasweet—a trade name for aspartame, an artificial sweetener

Oral glucose tolerance test (OGTT)—a medical test where you are asked to drink a glass of glucose quickly and then have your blood glucose tested several times over the next few hours to see how high your blood glucose goes

Orlistat—a drug that prevents the absorption of fat from your guts and is used to treat obesity

Osteoarthritis—a medical condition resulting in pain and stiffness in several bones and joints

Oxidative stress—a chemical reaction that can damage tissue in your body

Pancreatitis—a medical condition causing inflammation of the pancreas

Papaverine—a drug used to treat erectile dysfunction

Partial lipodystrophy—a rare medical condition associated with severe insulin resistance

Peritoneal dialysis—a medical procedure to filter impurities out of the body by putting liquid into the abdomen of someone whose kidneys are failing

Phentermine—a drug used to curb appetite

Phentolamine—a drug used to treat erectile dysfunction

Phenytoin—a drug used to treat seizure disorders and the pain from nerve damage

Phosphodiesterase-5-inhibitor—a class of drug used to treat erectile dysfunction

Pioglitazone—a drug used to treat insulin resistance

Pneumococcal pneumonia—a serious infection of the lungs caused by a bacterium

Polycystic ovarian syndrome (PCOS)—a medical condition in women that can cause insulin resistance

Pramlintide—a drug which is a long-acting analog of the hormone amylin, and which is used to treat type 1 diabetes

Prandin—a trade name for repaglinide, a drug used to increase insulin production

Pravachol—a trade name for pravastatin, a drug used to treat high cholesterol

Pravastatin—a drug used to treat high cholesterol

Precose—a trade name for acarbose, a drug that slows down the absorption of complex carbohydrates from your guts

Prediabetes—a medical term that is sometimes used to describe people who do not yet have diabetes but who are at high risk of getting diabetes in the future

Pregabalin—a drug used to treat the pain from damaged nerves

Pres Tab—a trade name for glyburide, a drug used to increase insulin production

Priapism—a medical condition where a man has a prolonged and painful erection

Proinsulin—the molecule that is formed when insulin and C-peptide are joined together

Prolactin—a hormone made in the pituitary gland in the brain

Protamine—a fish protein that is added to insulin to make it more long-acting

Prozac—a trade name for fluoxetine, a drug used to treat depression

Questran—a trade name for cholestyramine, a drug used to treat high cholesterol

Ramipril—an ACE-inhibitor drug used to lower blood pressure, protect the kidneys, and reduce the risk of heart disease

Rebound hyperglycemia—the idea that a low blood glucose can produce such a vigorous release of hormones that the blood glucose will rebound to very high levels

Redux—a trade name for dexfenfluramine, a drug used to curb appetite

Reglan—a trade name for metoclopramide, a drug used to treat nausea and gastroparesis

Repaglinide—a drug used to increase insulin production

Rezulin—a trade name for troglitazone, a drug that was used to treat insulin resistance but was taken off the market because it caused severe liver damage in some people

Riomet—a trade name for metformin, a drug used to treat insulin resistance

Rosiglitazone—a drug used to treat insulin resistance

Sertraline—a drug used to treat depression

"Sharps" container—a plastic box in which to safely dispose of needles and syringes

Sildenafil—a drug used to treat erectile dysfunction

Sitagliptin—a drug used to lower blood glucose

Starlix—a trade name for nateglinide, a drug used to increase insulin production

Statin drug—a class of drug used to treat high cholesterol

Somogyi phenomenon—an erroneous theory that high blood glucose levels are caused by an exaggerated "rebound" from a low blood glucose level

Symlin—a trade name for pramlintide, a drug used to help lower blood glucose in people with type 1 diabetes

Tadalafil—a drug used to treat erectile dysfunction

Thiazide diuretic—a class of drug used to lower blood pressure

Tolbutamide—a drug used to increase insulin production

Tolinase—a trade name for tolbutamide, a drug used to increase insulin production

Troglitazone—a drug that was used to treat insulin resistance but was taken off the market because it caused severe liver damage in some people

Type 1 diabetes—a type of diabetes that is more common in younger people, caused by the person's own immune system destroying the cells that make insulin

Type 2 diabetes—a type of diabetes that is more common in older people, caused by the progressive loss of insulin production and increased resistance to insulin

Type one-and-a-half diabetes—a sloppy term for diabetes that doctors and scientists find hard to classify

Uric acid—a chemical waste product which, if it builds up in your body, causes gout

Vanadium—a heavy metal element which mimics some of the things that insulin does and is sold as a "natural" supplement to help lower blood glucose

Vardenafil—a drug used to treat erectile dysfunction

Varenicline—a drug used to treat tobacco addiction

Viagra—a trade name for sildenafil, a drug used to treat erectile dysfunction

Wellbutrin—a trade name for bupropion, a drug used to treat tobacco addiction

Xenical—a trade name for orlistat, a drug that blocks fat absorption from your guts and is used to treat obesity

Zetia—a trade name for ezitimibe, a drug used to treat high cholesterol

Zocor—a trade name for simvastatin, a drug used to treat high cholesterol

Zoloft—a trade name for sertraline, a drug used to treat depression

Zyban—a trade name for bupropion, a drug used to treat tobacco addiction

Index

D

E

F

G

J

K

L

M

N

O

P

Q

R

S

T

About the Author

David K. McCulloch is a clinical professor of medicine at the University of Washington in Seattle. He has worked in the field of clinical diabetes innovation for over thirty years and has over eighty publications on a wide variety of diabetes-related topics. Since 1994, he has been the senior diabetes specialist at Group Health Cooperative, a health-care organization in Washington State with over half a million enrolled members.